THE INTEGRATED PRACTITIONER

Turning Tyrants into Tools in Health Practice

BOOK 3 OF *THE INTEGRATED PRACTITIONER* SERIES

JUSTIN AMERY

Radcliffe Publishing
London • New York

Radcliffe Publishing Ltd
St Mark's House
Shepherdess Walk
London N1 7LH
United Kingdom

www.radcliffehealth.com

British Library Cataloguing in Publication Data

A catalogue record for this book is available from the British Library.

ISBN-13: 978 184619 773 4
Volume set ISBN-13: 978 184619 950 9

The paper used for the text pages of this book is FSC® certified. FSC (The Forest Stewardship Council®) is an international network to promote responsible management of the world's forests.

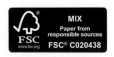

Typeset and designed by Darkriver Design, Auckland, New Zealand
Printed and bound by Hobbs the Printers, Totton, Hants, UK

Contents

About the author   vii

Acknowledgements   viii

Introduction to the series   1
- Why are these workbooks needed?   1
- Why did I write them?   2
- What will be in them?   3
- What perspectives and approaches will they use?   4
- Points and prizes: something for nothing   9
- Provisos   9

Chapter 1: The perspective of 'other'   11
- Tools or tyrants?   13

Chapter 2: Health knowledge   17
- A brief word of warning   17
- What do we know about health?   18
- Health as a relational entity   20
- Choosing what we see   20
- Testing our truths   22
- Knowledge and power   23
- Why is this important to health practice?   24

Chapter 3: Health beliefs   27
- Health beliefs and explanatory models   28
- Using explanatory models skilfully   33
- Conflicts and dissonance   34
- Integrating cultures and beliefs into our practice   36

Chapter 4: Information and guidelines   39
- The information explosion   40
- The effect of the information explosion in practice   41
- Guidelines   43
- Integrating information and guidelines into our practice   45

Contents

Chapter 5: Time and resources   47
- The problem of 'fairness'   48
- Practitioners, not priests   48
- The big (and small) issues   49
- Prioritising and choosing   50
- Mindful dedication   52
- Being firm about what we cannot do   54
- Acting effectively   56

Chapter 6: Regulations and targets   59
- Targets   61
- Integrating regulations and targets into our practice   63

Chapter 7: Organisations and teams   65
- Organisations as tools and tyrants   66
- Motivation   66
- The functions of health organisations   68
- Dysfunctional organisations   68
- Assessing our organisations   71
- How can we help our organisations work more effectively?   73
- Integrating organisations and teams   74

Chapter 8: Space and the environment   77
- What does our space say?   78
- Changes in health practice space   78
- Therapeutic environments   80
- Making consulting space more therapeutic   80
- Making hospital environments more therapeutic   82
- Integrating our space into our practice   84

Chapter 9: 'Effectiveness'   87
- How do we assess effectiveness?   89
- An empirical enquiry of effectiveness   90
- An interpretive enquiry of effectiveness   92
- Looking for 'evidence' of effectiveness   94
- Being wary of power claims dressed as knowledge claims   95
- Integrating and balancing approaches to health practice   96

Conclusion: integrated harmonic balance with the other   99
- The 'other' as tyrants   99
- The crucial importance (and power) of 'me'   99
- Integrating the 'other' into our practice   101

Notes 105

Bibliography 128

These books are dedicated to my Dad, Tony Amery, who was a wonderful doctor and who is still my inspiration.

About the author

I am a full-time practising family practitioner and children's palliative care specialist doctor working in the UK. I have also spent some years working in Uganda and other sub-Saharan African countries.

I enjoy teaching, writing and mentoring. I am a medical student tutor at the University of Oxford, a trainer in general practice, and I have designed and set up children's palliative care courses for health professionals in the UK and Africa. I have worked with 'failing practices' to help them turn round; and also with health professionals who are struggling (as we all do from time to time).

I have always had an interest in philosophy and spirituality, and have studied this at postgraduate level. I have carried out some research into education and training of health professionals around the world and I continue to explore that interest.

I have previously written two books: *Children's Palliative Care in Africa* (Oxford: Oxford University Press, 2009) and the Association for Children's Palliative Care (ACT) *Handbook of Children's Palliative Care for GPs* (Bristol: ACT, 2011). I particularly enjoy reading and writing poetry.

At heart, though, I am a practitioner and a generalist. What is more, as you can probably see, I am rather a jack of all trades, and a master of none.

I have been motivated to write this book as I am hoping to explore practical ways of practising health that help us all, patients and practitioners alike, to become a little more healthy, and a little more whole.

Acknowledgements

These books have been brewing up over many years and so there have been very, very many influences upon them. There are far too many people to mention and thank without risking leaving someone out, so I shall just mention those who have been immediately involved.

Firstly, thank you to those very kind and patient people who helped review the drafts and gave such helpful feedback: Maria Ward, Penny Thompson, Meriel Lynch, Tom Nicholson-Lailey, Peter Burke, Penny Moore, Susan McCrae, Caitlin Chasser, Louise Rutter, Polly Steele, Rachel Samson, Laura Ingle and Maddy Podichetty.

I would also particularly like to mention Chris Smith, who not only gave very useful feedback on these books, but who also helped me to develop a lot of the ideas in them through his leadership of the Oxford Advanced Consultation Skills Course that I help him with, and over a few pints in the pub as well.

Thanks as well to Gillian Nineham of Radcliffe Publishing, who was brave (or daft) enough to put her faith in these rather unconventional offerings; suggest numerous areas for improvement and offer tremendous support and encouragement in their publication. Thanks also to Jamie Etherington and Camille Lowe for all their help in putting them together.

I would like to thank my colleagues at Bury Knowle Health Centre in Oxford, Helen House Hospice in Oxford, Hospice Africa in Kampala, Uganda, and Keech Hospice in Luton. They have all shown utmost patience and perseverance as I have led them on various merry dances, contortions and deviations in the name of 'good ideas', rarely reminding me of the 99% which failed, and always supportive of the 1% that, miraculously, did.

Of course I can't forget Karen Bateman (the doctor) and Karen Amery (the missus) who has been a continuous and never-ending source of sound advice, support and wisdom.

Finally, I would like to offer a huge thank you to Polly who, on a cliff top in Spain, gave me the courage to risk writing this stuff down and making it public.

Introduction to the series

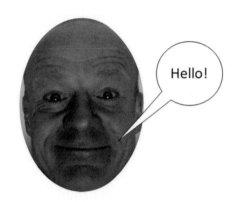

Hello!

Hello and welcome! This is me. You and I will be sharing a journey through this book, so you may wish to know what I look like. Because practice can't happen without practitioners, I will be popping up now and again, to test-drive some of the ideas that we will be discussing.

WHY ARE THESE WORKBOOKS NEEDED?

If you are, like me, a modern-day practitioner, you are probably still dedicated to the idea of good practice, but feeling rather buffeted by many and various winds of change that are sweeping through. You are also probably feeling (like me) that it would be good to have two minutes to sit back and reflect a little: to think about what's working and what's not; and maybe even to find a little balance.

If this is how you feel, you have come to the right place. So welcome!

In this series of workbooks we will be doing exactly that, taking a little time out, thinking about what we are doing, looking at things from different perspectives and using different lenses, and trying out some practical ways of making our practice more effective, more efficient, and (above all) more satisfying.

On the other hand . . .

If you are, like me, a modern-day practitioner, you will probably also be moving far too quickly to have any time for doing anything except what you need to be doing. In other words, you probably don't feel you have time for luxuries like sitting back and thinking. Frustrating though it may be, you probably have time to do only what you *have* to do, rather than what you *want* to do.

If this is how you feel, you are still in the right place, so welcome again!

In this series of workbooks, we will be working under the clock, recognising that there are boxes to tick and targets to hit. No doubt you don't just need to keep up to date, you need to prove you are keeping up to date too, for appraisal, or for review, or for revalidation. So, as we go along, we will be providing practical examples that will help you not just to reflect upon but actually to develop your practice.

What's more, we will even be providing appraisal certificates, so our appraisers, line managers and bosses will stay happy too!

But you're gonna have to serve somebody, yes indeed
You're gonna have to serve somebody,
Well, it may be the devil or it may be the Lord
But you're gonna have to serve somebody.

– Bob Dylan

WHY DID I WRITE THEM?

I have written these workbooks because there doesn't seem to be anything out there that scratches my itch. Our experience of real-life health practice is messy, complex and often chaotic. It doesn't seem to bear much resemblance to the practice we read about, or even the practice we try to teach our students and trainees.

Modern scientific and philosophical understandings of the universe are complex, messy and relational too. But our models of health and health practice often seem to be built on glib and simplistic models, or they fall into dualistic discussions (for example, about 'patient-centred' or 'practitioner-centred' care; or about 'traditional' or 'alternative' practice; or even about 'disease' and 'health'). Is the world really like that?

I have also written these books as I am worried about the levels of demoralisation and burnout among students, trainees and colleagues that I meet, right across the globe. Of course we can all get a bit tired, burnt out, and maybe even ill. If we are honest, we are often sceptical and occasionally a little cynical about what we do. But if we are even more honest than that, at heart we believe in what we do, because we think it is important.

It's not that we want to turn the clock back. We can feel a considerable (if quiet) sense of pride in how far health practice has developed. But perhaps we'd also like to think that, in the 21st century, there is a way for our practice to include and yet somehow to transcend what has gone before. It's not that we want to reject the practicalities, the science, the technology and the politics. On the contrary, I think most of us wish to accept and value them. But we also want to do what evolution always does: including, building upon and then transcending what has gone before. In so doing, maybe we can also rediscover the art of what we do, and perhaps even find a way of expressing ourselves with a little more poetry.

WHAT WILL BE IN THEM?

The answer to that is simple really. We are hoping to look at practice from different perspectives, and using different lenses, so each book takes a different view.

- Workbook 1 – *Surviving and Thriving in Health Practice*. We are the foundation of everything we do. Without us there would be no health practice. We are our own most useful tools. So, in the first book, we will look at how we can keep ourselves sharp, surviving and thriving in practice.

- Workbook 2 – *Co-creating in Health Practice*. As practitioners, whenever we come into contact with our patients, we create something very familiar but also very strange: a relationship. This relationship is neither me nor the patient, but some sort of third entity, which has an existence of its own, partly from me, and partly from the patient. This 'co-creation' is arguably our most powerful tool, but it is a tricky one to use. So we will focus on that in the second workbook, considering how we might practise in a way that co-creates healthier and happier existences, for both our patients and ourselves.

- Workbook 3 – *Turning Tyrants into Tools in Health Practice*. As practitioners we have a vast array of tools that we can use: time, computers, money, information, colleagues, equipment, targets, our workplaces and so on. If they get out of balance, however, each of these tools can become a tyrant, so that it has control of us, rather than the other way round. So in workbook 3 we will be looking at some of the most important tools (and tyrants), considering how we can stay in control of them (and not vice versa).

- Workbook 4 – *Integrating Everything*. Health practice is, ultimately, a single integrated thing. While workbooks 1–3 have been looking at the different 'bits' of this 'whole', workbook 4 is where the rubber hits the road, because it is here that we try to put it all together and come up with ways that we can integrate everything into a happier, healthier and more skilful whole within the real-life, complex and messy world of health practice.

- Workbook 5 – *Food for Thought*. We are practitioners, so we are practical, and interested in practice. So we will leave the theory until last. But most of us like a little bit of theoretical background to give context to, and to underpin our practice.[1] So workbook 5 tries to provide that. Everything that exists does so against a background. Indeed the word 'exist' means to 'stand out'. All of our experiences, beliefs and understandings of health practice derive from a living, organic and constantly moving context: whether scientific, philosophical, cultural, aesthetic, biological or spiritual. It is useful therefore to spend a little time understanding and reflecting on these building blocks of who we are. As practitioners, we don't always have time to do this, so we will leave this book until last. It will be a little luxury for those with a little more time, not essential, but hopefully a bit nourishing. Like a fireside cup of cocoa.

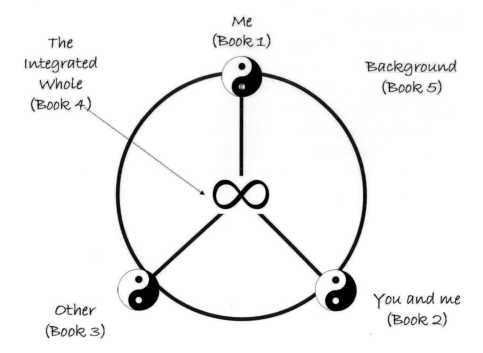

WHAT PERSPECTIVES AND APPROACHES WILL THEY USE?

In the 21st century we practise healthcare in a strange tension.

Science has taught us that we live in a highly relational, messy, multidimensional, complex, blurry and even chaotic universe. The humanities and philosophy have taught us that much of what we hold to be 'true' is relational and cultural and socially constructed. The arts teach us the value of creativity and expression in all walks of life. Spirituality teaches us about perspective, the value of awareness, and the fundamental interconnectedness of all things.

However, despite this relationality, creativity and complexity, we seem to be practising in a world that seems ever more bound and codified, with ever more targets and tick boxes, according to models that seem unrealistically geometric and two-dimensional, and with ever less room to breathe and to express ourselves.

So, in these workbooks, we will try to be practical and pragmatic. While we may not necessarily like the rules, regulations, guidelines, laws and targets that have nosed into our practice, we recognise that they have their uses. We know that health is a political football, and we are used to being kicked around a bit.

As practitioners in the 21st century we also value (and sometimes worry about) the advances that science and technology have brought. As practitioners, we are scientists, and we have a duty to do our best to ensure that what we do is as safe and effective as possible. We recognise that finding an evidence base for what we do is important not just for safety, but for development too.

So in these workbooks, we will start from the premise that we should, wherever possible, look for empirical evidence for what we are suggesting. On the other hand, we will remain vigilant to the blind spots of the empirical and technological approach, and look for alternatives to fill any gaps that we find.

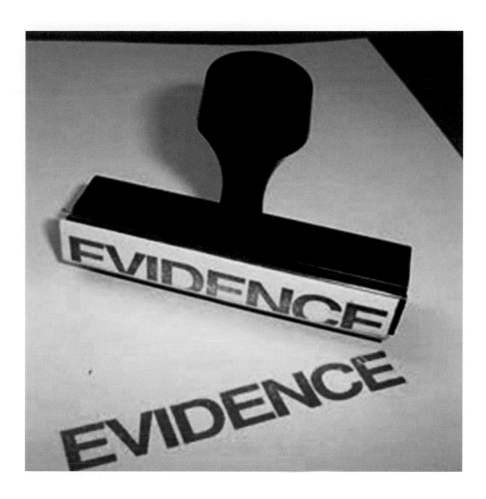

Wherever possible we will look for empirical evidence for what we are suggesting.

As modern practitioners we are scientists, and also technicians, but we are artists too. There is an art to being a practitioner, and in fact practice is an art. We might lose sight of it sometimes, but we are in the business (and busy-ness) of trying to create healthier and happier existences for our patients, and hopefully for ourselves too.

So in these workbooks we will be using plenty of imagery, art and illustration to engage the more creative sides of our brains, and to remind us that integrated practitioners need to be able to find balance between creative and practical.

These days, we don't tend to talk much about spirituality. Many of us would not think of ourselves as 'religious', and some of us might be horrified at the idea that modern-day practice should have anything to do with spirituality.

But most of us perhaps like to feel that there is some purpose or meaning behind what we do. We may hope that our practice connects with and somehow reflects the values and traditions of our families as well as of our broader societies and cultures. We deal with life and death, and so with the many existential and spiritual questions that arise as a consequence. If we are to be integrated practitioners, we need to have a handle on these too.

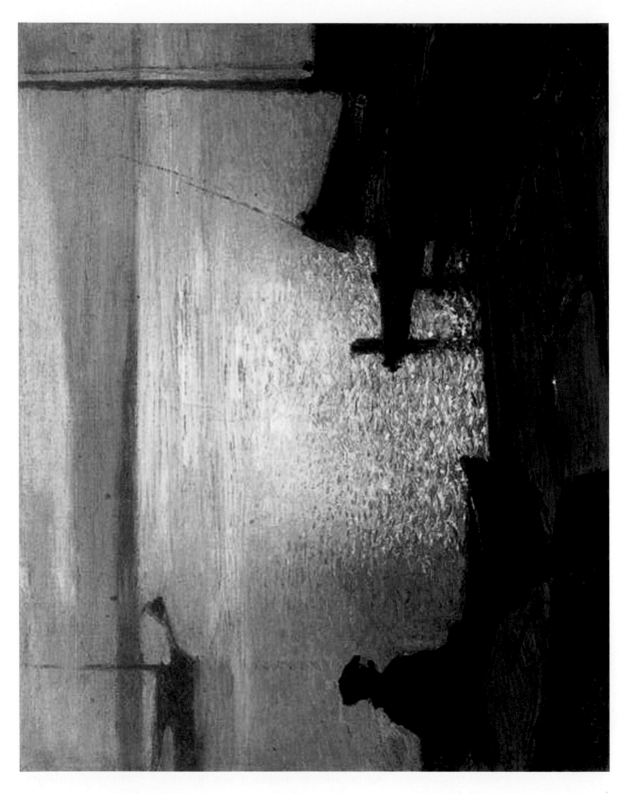

'Along the Mystic River' – for some reason I have found myself drawn to rivers as I have written this book, so a few will be popping up as we go along.[2]

So, in these workbooks we will try to look around the edges and to peer through the gaps, asking not just: 'What should we do?' but also 'Why should we do it?' and 'What does it all mean anyway?'

Finally, we don't have to practise long to realise that there are some things that make no sense, and from which no sense can be made. Random and chaotic events, reactions and emotions may arise, surprisingly. These can be both deeply troubling but also deeply wonderful, in that they can give expression to the inexpressible. We practitioners are practical people. We like to 'do' things. But sometimes there is nothing we can do, because there is nothing to be done. At these times, we have to just 'be'. For just 'being', for making sense of nonsense, and for making nonsense of sense, there is nothing better than poetry. So we will be seeing a fair bit of that too.

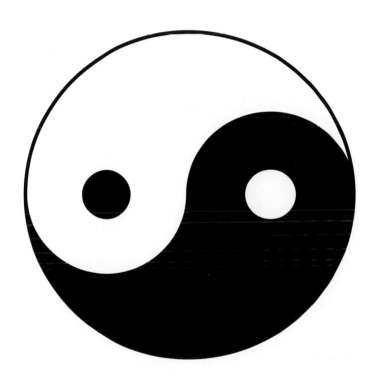

Symbols and rituals are fascinating things that in some way speak to us at a 'level beyond'. It is not often easy to make sense of them, and yet we may be surprised to find that our practice is full of them.

Ars Poetica

A poem should be palpable and mute
As a globed fruit,
Dumb
As old medallions to the thumb,
Silent as the sleeve-worn stone
Of casement ledges where the moss has grow –
A poem should be wordless
As the flight of birds.
*

A poem should be motionless in time
As the moon climbs,
Leaving, as the moon releases
Twig by twig the night-entangled trees,
Leaving, as the moon behind the winter leaves.
Memory by memory the mind–
A poem should be motionless in time
As the moon climbs.
*

A poem should be equal to:
Not true.
For all the history of grief
An empty doorway and a maple leaf.
For love
The leaning grasses and two lights above the sea–
A poem should not mean
But be.

– Archibald MacLeish[3]

POINTS AND PRIZES: SOMETHING FOR NOTHING

In the initial stages of this book, my publisher explained that medical publishing is at a turning point. Whereas before practitioners might choose a book that they would enjoy reading, nowadays they are too busy for that. So the upshot is that we only read books we need to read, rather than those we want to read.

A bit like Nanny McPhee . . .

The good news about adopting an integrated approach is we don't need to judge, we just need to adapt. If that is the way of the world, so be it, and so we have.

The particular way of the current world of health practice (at least where I currently work in the UK) appears to be a focus on objectives, outcomes, points and prizes. So the initial book has been adapted to match. Each chapter will contain activities and reflections that will meet common curriculum areas for medical and nursing practice. At the end of each book is a link to the Radcliffe Continuing Professional Development site, www.radcliffehealth.com/cpd, where you can download certificates that you can use for your CPD, appraisal or revalidation requirements.

OK, I admit it's a bit tongue in cheek, but there's no rule to say that we can't have fun while toeing the line, is there?

PROVISOS

I am, at heart, a practitioner, and a general practitioner at that. That means I am a bit of a jack of all trades, but master of none. I am partial, biased and subjective. The book is intended for all health practitioners but, inevitably, and despite my best efforts, no doubt the 'male', 'medical' and 'Western' nature of my experiences and thoughts will peep through. I hope you feel able to forgive them and look past them.

Also, I can quite honestly say that there is nothing new in this book, and I doubt there is anything in it that you could not find better argued and more coherently evidenced in other places. There is some philosophy, science, spirituality, art and poetry, but I am not a philosopher, scientist, guru, artist or poet. I am a health practitioner who dabbles.

So I have referenced those sources I can remember and can find. Others may be lost in the mists. But I do not claim any of the basic ideas in this book as my own. I have simply looked at them from my personal perspective and tried to put them together in a way that I have found useful in my own practice and in my own teaching. I hope you can enjoy them, and that you will forgive the numerous mistakes and omissions that you will undoubtedly find.

Chapter 1
The perspective of 'other'

Activity 1.1: Tools (30 minutes)

Take a few minutes to reflect on your practice.

List down all of the different people or entities that you need in order to be able to practise effectively.

Don't just think about physical objects, like stethoscopes or pens, but think very broadly. For example, what about time and space, or laws, or money?

In the last two workbooks, we have been looking at the 'human' elements of health practice. Many health practitioners are 'people people', so the first two workbooks will probably have been fairly easy reading. This workbook is about some of the important non-human entities that we need in order to practise. Therefore, for 'people people', this workbook may seem a little drier and take a little bit more concentration, but it is crucial to the attempt to become an integrated practitioner, so please read on.

In order to provide integrated healthcare, we need to integrate a huge number of 'other' external entities; for example, time, space, information, equipment, colleagues, regulations, guidelines, drugs and money. We also have to draw on less tangible 'other' internal entities, such as our knowledge, understanding, language, values and beliefs.

Each one of these entities can be a useful tool for our practice. To be effective practitioners, we hope to gain some mastery of them. But sometimes we feel as if they have mastery of us.

There are days when we feel on top of our game, we keep to time, we know

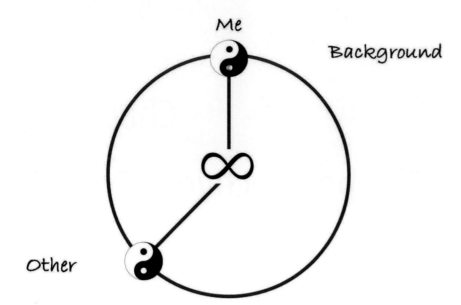

Me

Background

Other

In practice key relationships are with
ourselves and with our patients,
but there are many, many 'other'
entities with whom we are in
relationship too.

instantly what's wrong, the right treatment is immediately to hand, our colleagues
are supportive and helpful, and birdsong drifts through our open summer window.

Then there are the other days . . .

Research shows the same picture the whole world over: only a fraction of our time
is spent with patients; and only a fraction of that fraction is spent truly connecting,
listening and responding.[4]

> Although we think of the patient as the main focus of our practice, often
> we can lose this focus under the barrage of all these 'other' factors, and even
> become stressed or unwell as a result of them. The life of a modern health
> practitioner often feels like plate-spinning gone mad. What is more, our
> plate-spinning, juggling act takes place within apparently ever-tightening
> constraints: time, money, space, targets, guidelines, regulation, ethics,
> knowledge, and so on.

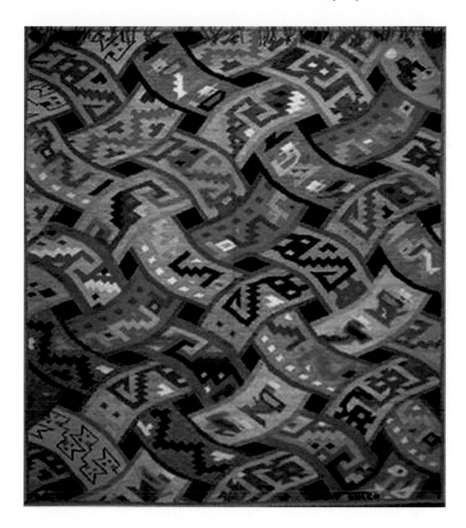

As practitioners we have to weave together a huge number of disparate strands to create an integrated whole. (Photo of 'Weaving the Weave' by master weaver Edwin Sulca Lagos[5])

TOOLS OR TYRANTS?

As integrated practitioners, we hope to find, balance and integrate all the 'other' entities that are of most relevance and use at that moment, and exclude those that are not of use, so that our practice is one integrated and balanced process, tailored to the needs of the patient and the moment.

When used skilfully, our tools become an aid to effective practice. However, if we are not careful, our tools can also assume a magnified importance, becoming ends in themselves.

This is when tools become tyrants.[6]

For example, we may focus too much on time at the expense of our patients (or vice versa); or we may focus too much on the acquisition of theoretical knowledge and insufficiently on the application of that knowledge in practice (or vice versa); or we may focus too much on our own values and beliefs and insufficiently on the values and beliefs of our patients and colleagues (or vice versa); or we may focus too much on organisational and government targets and objectives and insufficiently on considering the needs of the patient (or vice versa).

If we can achieve a healthy 'me', and work in a healthy team, a healthy organisation, a healthy environment, within a realistic time-frame, according to values, rules and ethics that we can own and share, using thoroughly acquired and relevant knowledge, skills and competencies, and with adequate resources, then we have a good chance of being 'good enough' (and happy) practitioners.

On the other hand, if we work out of an unhealthy 'me'; within a dysfunctional team and organisation, in a cluttered and chaotic space, constantly running late, according to rules, values and ethics that we cannot accept or buy into, without sufficient knowledge, skills and competencies, and with inadequate resources, then it is unlikely we will be able to be even good-enough practitioners, and we will probably be less happy in our practice.

So, in the remainder of this book, we will spend some time looking at some of the factors that researchers have shown to have the greatest impact (positive or negative) on health practice and health practitioners. For each, we shall try to find ways of mastering them as tools, stopping them becoming tyrants, and integrating them in a harmonically balanced way into our practice.

Activity 1.2: Tyrants (30 minutes)

Reflect on the list you drew up in Activity 1.1. Consider which of these entities or people you have control over, and which have control over you. Take a little more time and start to consider which of these may not just have control over you, but in fact may be oppressing you in some way. Perhaps they generate a sense of fear or dislike or tension when you think about them, or you worry about them before, during or after your practice.

Now start to rank these entities or people in order: from the most tyrannical to the least.

The night is darkening round me

The night is darkening round me,
The wild winds coldly blow;
But a tyrant spell has bound me,
And I cannot, cannot go.

The giant trees are bending
Their bare boughs weighed with snow;
The storm is fast descending,
And yet I cannot go.

Clouds beyond clouds above me,
Wastes beyond wastes below;
But nothing drear can move me;
I will not, cannot go.

— Emily Jane Brontë

Chapter 2
Health knowledge

Activity 2.1: Reflection on health (30 minutes)

How do you feel now? Would you say you feel 'healthy' or 'unhealthy'?

Either way, could you define exactly what you mean?

Even if you feel 'healthy', are there 'parts' of you that still feel 'unhealthy'?

What about vice versa?

A BRIEF WORD OF WARNING

At first sight this might appear rather an odd and confusing chapter, because it is going to demonstrate that we don't know much of what we think we know, even about health (about which we probably think we know a lot).

If you are not of a philosophical persuasion, you can skip it, and move straight to the next chapter, on health beliefs. You won't miss anything crucial.

But just make sure you leave your certainties behind. You won't need them from here on in.

WHAT DO WE KNOW ABOUT HEALTH?

As practitioners, we probably think that we know a fair bit about health, and that most of what we know is true.

If so, before we go any further in this book, we may need to think again.

Consider this statement: 'This statement is false.'

This is a statement that can be neither true nor false. If it is false, it is true. If it is true, it is false. The key to the paradox are the words 'this statement'. The statement refers to itself for its own definition. It is a 'self-referential' statement.

The problem with all 'truths' to which we ascribe 'meaning' is that the truth, meaning and expression of those truths and meanings (through thought and language) are part of the same 'self-referential' system.[7] Self-referential logical systems always end up in paradox (Gödel's theorem[8]).

Have a look at the endnotes if you'd like to explore this strange but crucial idea in more detail. In simple terms, though, we can't really 'know' what 'truth' is.

To illustrate this point, think of these three interconnected entities: thought, language and meaning. Does thought generate language or does language generate thought? Is there such a thing as language without meaning, or meaning without language? Can truth have no meaning, or meaning have no truth? Does truth exist if it cannot be expressed through language or thought?

Wherever we start on this cycle, we find ourselves caught in a paradoxical loop, unable to define one entity without recourse to another in the same loop.

Health has no independent existence. We can point at health or wave at it. It exists partly as an idea or thought, partly as a meaning we can express through language and partly as a behaviour we can display. Because 'health' is a form of 'truth', and also an idea that we can hold to have meaning and also express through language, it is part of its own self-referential loop. Logically therefore, we have to accept we can't ever really 'know' what 'health' 'is' either.

That's a strange state of affairs for health practitioners, isn't it?

Well, not really. If we live in a relational and interdependent universe, perhaps we shouldn't be surprised to find our beliefs and knowledge are relational and interdependent too, and that at the heart of truth is paradox.

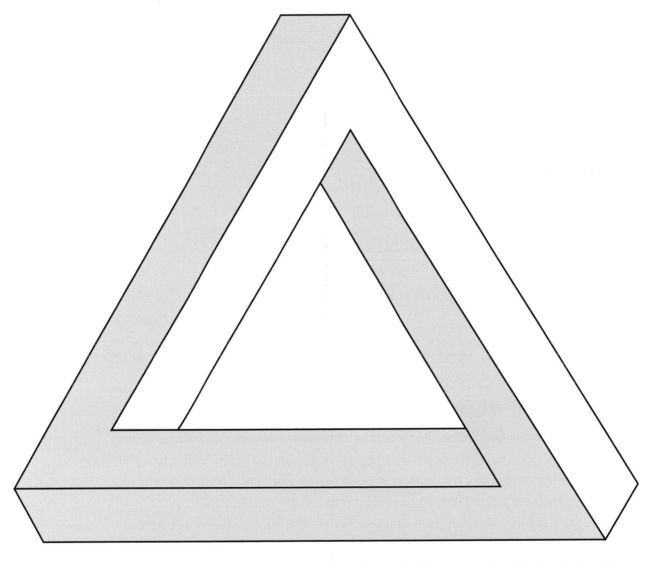

The Penrose Triangle – a visual form of self-referential paradox. Each angle looks fine, because our mind 'refers' to the two three-dimensional lines that make the angle. As a whole, the shape becomes impossible, because our mind refers outside of the shape to realise that it can't 'work' in practice. So three possible angles make an impossible shape. This is an example of paradox arising out of 'self-reference'.

HEALTH AS A RELATIONAL ENTITY

If you are feeling increasingly unsettled, you are not alone. Discovering the fundamental paradox and uncertainty at the heart of our practice is quite hard to swallow.

However, we might also feel that we have a duty to ourselves and our patients to give this serious thought. As practitioners patients come to us to seek for truths about their health, as well as for help with managing it.

If we are not aware of the relativity and paradox behind the truths we believe to be true, how can we help our patients find truths about their health that are effective and make sense for them?

If we are not aware that we are aiming for a nebulous and shifting thing, we might get frustrated and demoralised that we never seem to be able to arrive at our goal, that it stays, agonisingly, always just out of reach . . .

seeker of truth

seeker of truth

follow no path

all paths lead where

truth is here

— e. e. cummings[9]

CHOOSING WHAT WE SEE

There is another very good reason to be cautious about what we hold to be 'true' about health. This is because what we believe about truths automatically influences the way we look for them, which in turn dictates what we find, and so reinforces what we believe. In other words, we tend to find the truths we look for.

If we look 'inside',[10] we will find different forms of truth compared to when we look at the 'outside'.[11] If we look from the perspective of the individual, we will find different truths compared to if we look from the perspective of family, culture or society.[12] If we choose to be deductive we will arrive at different destinations than if we choose to be inductive or creative, and either approach can leave as many questions as answers.[13] There are many ways of 'knowing', none of which appears to be perfect in all situations.[14]

So if we believe health to be a certain thing, we tend to choose ways of viewing and practising it which make it more likely we will experience it in ways that match our beliefs, and become blind to ways that challenge our beliefs. Blindness is rarely a helpful quality in health practitioners.

If we are not mindfully aware of the fundamental uncertainty of our beliefs, we may become stuck in a closed-minded loop, which may shut out alternative and possibly more effective perspectives about what truths like 'health' might 'be'.

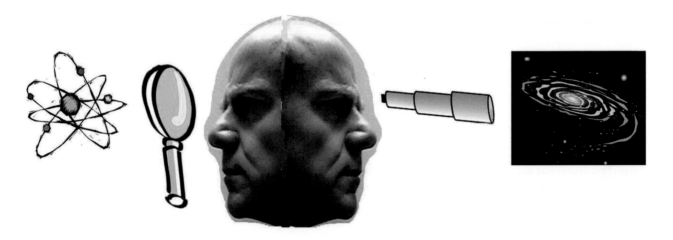

Rather strangely, choosing the way we look determines what truths we might find.

Activity 2.2: Group-think (15 minutes)

Think of any health condition, say, for example, schizophrenia.

Think back into the history of health practice over the last thousand years or so. What different 'truths' have health practitioners held about that condition? For example, spiritual, criminal, psychological, molecular, biological, cultural, societal?

Which of these 'truths' about schizophrenia would you say have been more or less 'effective'?

Think a bit more. Why did a particular group interpretation shift into another one? Was it because health practitioners at the time realised they were 'wrong', or was it that alternative discoveries, technologies and understandings shifted whole world views of those groups of practitioners at those times?

Now think forward a thousand years. Do you think we have reached the limit of truth about health? If not, what 'truths' that we currently hold about health will we (or our successors) be eventually looking back on in horror?

TESTING OUR TRUTHS

We can always test our truths. But it makes no sense to use the wrong test for the particular truth claim we are making. Scientific (empirical) testing will be very helpful to test a drug company's truth claims about the safety and efficacy of a new drug, whereas metaphysical tools will not. However, scientific testing will not be helpful to test the validity of a patient's claim that she feels hopeless; or of a society's claim that drug addiction is a disease rather than a crime.

Choosing the wrong test for the claim in hand is a mistake we often fall into as practitioners. It is easy to take one perspective, and try to squeeze all truth claims into it. We sometimes even set things up in opposition. For example, we often hear people ask: 'Is practice an art or a science?' Of course it is both, and more. Being an integrated practitioner means becoming aware of and being able to use all of these different forms of knowledge, and choosing the most effective tool for the particular patient and context.

Activity 2.3: Your own perspective and practice (30 minutes)

Take a quiet moment and reflect peacefully on your own health practice. Of the different sorts of knowledge outlined above, which ones have you been trained in and which do you tend to use?

How might these particular perspectives be influencing what you 'see' and how you practise?

Conversely, are there any ways they might blind you to other perspectives and practices that might be effective for your patients or for yourself?

KNOWLEDGE AND POWER

If this were just an academic argument, we would not include it in a practical work-book like this. But unfortunately these interesting theoretical observations have very significant practical implications, which can tyrannise both us and our patients.

That is because we don't make truth claims in a vacuum. We make truth claims because we hope to influence what we, or others (particularly our patients), 'ought' to do. Indeed, knowledge which does not tell us what we 'ought' to do may appear to be of limited use. However, this kind of 'prescriptive' knowledge is not really knowledge at all, as there is no logical link between what 'I know' and what 'you ought' to do.[15]

For this reason, we can view knowledge as a form of power, and knowledge claims as (at least partly), power claims.[16]

This is a very important insight for health practitioners, who are often called upon by patients to offer advice on what they 'ought' to do. As independent as we like to think we are, we cannot help being 'agents' of various interests and groups, such as the state, academia, religious groups, the bio-pharmaceutical industry, the complementary and alternative medicine industry, the bourgeoisie, or simply of our own vested interest.

> For example, with my family practitioner hat on I may often encourage peo-ple to stop smoking – a classical 'ought' statement. My 'reasoning' usually goes something like this (although hopefully with a little more gentle tact!)
> - You smoke – TRUE – this is an 'is' statement of fact (assuming the patient confesses!)
> - Smoking causes cancer – PROBABLY TRUE BUT DIFFICULT TO PROVE WITH 100% CERTAINTY. We can only say that empirical evidence strongly suggests that smoking causes cancer, and that the particular patient's chance of getting cancer rises significantly if he smokes.
> - So you ought to stop smoking – NOT TRUE. There is no logical connec-tion between the assertion that smoking appears to cause cancer and that the patient *ought* to stop. My claim that my patient should stop smoking is partly a power claim ('I know what is best for you') and is also partly influenced by subjective and self-interested influences (such as my medicalised view of health, the grounding belief that health is worth more than pleasure and the simple fact my pay is at least partly related to my success in stopping people smoking).

WHY IS THIS IMPORTANT TO HEALTH PRACTICE?

As health practitioners, we hope to have a broad and deep understanding of truths such as health. Knowledge such as this is an extremely powerful tool. But there is something more powerful still, because it affects the way we apply that knowledge. That something is wisdom, and at the heart of wisdom is the understanding that all truths are based on paradox and mystery.

The only true wisdom is in knowing you know nothing.

– Socrates

That is not to say we are stuck. There is much we can practically do. By being aware of the different forms of knowledge, and the appropriate form of enquiry for each different relationship and perspective, we can significantly broaden our skills as practitioners, using empirical, constructed and metaphysical approaches, and deductive or creative thinking as the situation demands.

In applying these different forms of knowledge, we can become more aware of the ultimate beliefs upon which we are basing our knowledge claims; and then use careful deductive logic to try to apply these knowledge claims as effectively as possible.

Exercising truth claims means exercising power. Power is something we cannot avoid having as health practitioners, because our patients are vulnerable. It can be very useful. But, if we are to be effective we hope to use it skilfully and compassionately, not unskilfully and tyrannically. That means we need to be mindfully aware of what 'truths' about 'health' we 'believe' to be 'true'.

In making knowledge claims about what patients (or students, or staff, or colleagues) 'ought' to do, we can also try to become more aware about what power claims we are simultaneously making, so that we can try to balance these claims as far towards the interests of our patients as we possibly can.

And, in order to guard against arrogance and complacency in our beliefs and practice, we may wish to keep in mind that ultimately, whatever we think we know, we know nothing.

All is Truth

O ME, *man of slack faith so long!*
Standing aloof—denying portions so long;
Only aware to-day of compact, all-diffused truth;
Discovering to-day there is no lie, or form of lie, and can be
  none, but grows as
inevitably
upon
itself as the truth does upon itself,
Or as any law of the earth, or any natural production of the
  earth does.

(This is curious, and may not be realized immediately—But
  it must be realized;
I feel in myself that I represent falsehoods equally with the
  rest,
And that the universe does.)

Where has fail'd a perfect return, indifferent of lies or the
  truth?
Is it upon the ground, or in water or fire? or in the spirit of
  man? or in the meat and
blood?

Meditating among liars, and retreating sternly into myself, I
  see that there are really no
liars or
lies after all,
And that nothing fails its perfect return—And that what are
  called lies are perfect
returns,
And that each thing exactly represents itself, and what has
  preceded it,

And that the truth includes all, and is compact, just as
  much as space is compact,
And that there is no flaw or vacuum in the amount of the
  truth—but that all is truth
without
exception;
And henceforth I will go celebrate anything I see or am,
And sing and laugh, and deny nothing.

– Walt Whitman

Chapter 3
Health beliefs

Health does not have any concrete existence. We can't see it passing by at the window. Its only existence is within our consciousness. All we can say about it is that it is a concept about which we have certain beliefs.

It is self-evident that if our beliefs about health are unhealthy, they will not be very helpful in our health practice. So what are our beliefs, and how do these beliefs affect our practice?

Are they tools or tyrants?

HEALTH BELIEFS AND EXPLANATORY MODELS

Individuals, families, societies and cultures have developed beliefs about 'health' and 'treatment' that makes sense to them, in their context, at their time. We are all the same in this, even though my beliefs might be quite different to yours. Just because we are health practitioners does not except us from this 'truth'. While we may have more knowledge *about* health than other people, our view of what health actually *is* remains only a belief, not a demonstrable fact. We can no more prove or disprove our beliefs than can our patients, our colleagues, or practitioners from different traditions or disciplines.

However, while our health beliefs may be hard to pin down, the out-workings of our health beliefs are very concrete, and have consequences, for better or for worse. Therefore the study of health beliefs is a very important one, which we might want to spend a few minutes thinking about.

The anthropological study of health belief is a fascinating one, and asks of different individuals, cultures and societies such questions as:

- What do you mean by the 'body'?
- How do you believe the body 'works'?
- How do you 'suffer' as individuals and as a whole culture and society?
- What is the 'mind' to you?
- What is the 'spirit' to you?
- What do perceptions such as 'pain' and 'well-being' mean to you?
- How do your health practitioners and patients interact?
- What is the role and status of your health practitioners?
- What is the role of nature, diet and nutrition for health?
- What chemicals and tools do you use to try to improve health?
- How has new information and new knowledge affected your health practices and beliefs?

To answer these questions, we each use 'explanatory models'.[17] Explanatory models describe our ideas and beliefs about what we mean by 'illness', the causes of illness, how we might 'diagnose' and how we might 'treat' illness.

Explanatory models are as diverse and infinite as humanity: for example, 'bio-medical', 'humoral', 'spiritual', 'psychological', 'naturopathic' or 'sociological' models.[18]

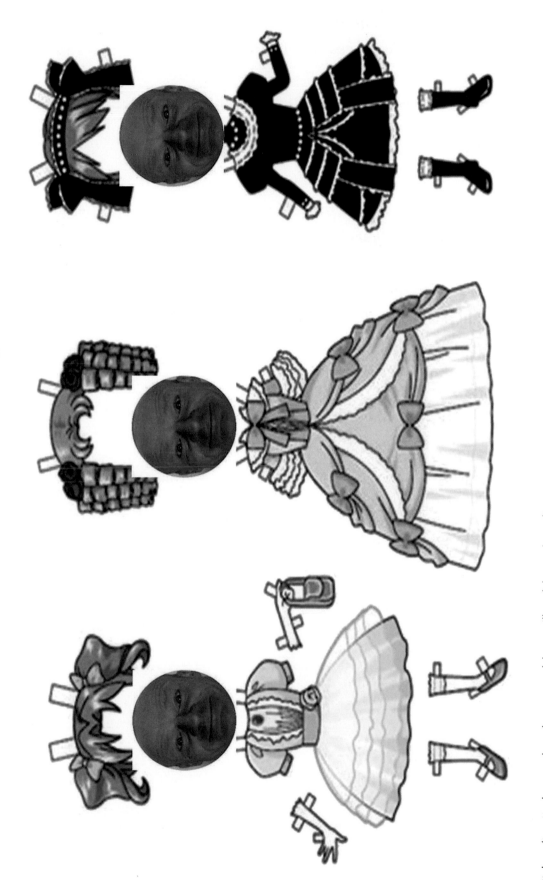

It doesn't matter how we dress them up. Models are still models, not the reality.

Spiritual Song of the Aborigine

I am a child of the Dreamtime People
Part of this Land, like the gnarled gumtree
I am the river, softly singing
Chanting our songs on my way to the sea
My spirit is the dust-devils
Mirages, that dance on the plain
I'm the snow, the wind and the falling rain
I'm part of the rocks and the red desert earth
Red as the blood that flows in my veins
I am eagle, crow and snake that glides
Thorough the rain-forest that clings to the mountainside
I awakened here when the earth was new
There was emu, wombat, kangaroo
No other man of a different hue
I am this land
And this land is me
I am Australia.

– Hyllus Maris[19]

In practice, we may hold more than one 'explanatory model' at any one time. Take me, for example:

> I am a Western-trained family doctor, with a special interest in children's palliative care. I have worked mainly in the UK, but also in various countries in Africa, particularly Uganda. I am schooled and practice primarily in the biomedical and psychological models. However, there are parts of the humoral, naturopathic and spiritual models that I find useful in practice.
>
> One of the trickiest decisions in any children's palliative care scenario is the decision about when to stop life-prolonging treatment. One of the reasons why it is so difficult is that it requires the coming together of different explanatory models. Here are three real-life (anonymised) dilemmas that I have had to work through. They illustrate quite well the issues that arise out of different explanatory models.
>
> - In the first case, I was working at a hospice in Oxford when a South Asian mother and her small child turned up unexpectedly at the front door. They had just got off the plane to the UK, where they hoped to get curative treatment for the child's cancer. They had initially gone to the local hospital who had told them to come to us. Although there were language barriers, it was clear enough from the assessment that the child had advanced, disseminated cancer, was in severe pain, and was close to death. We tried to explain this as best we could, and largely succeeded. The mother accepted that her child was dying. However, when it came to giving her child some pain relief, the mother refused it. She made clear that his pain was Karmic in origin and that, if he did not suffer it, he would still carry the karmic penalty into the next life. On those grounds, she refused treatment. After much ineffective discussion, including the involvement of a local Hindu priest, we eventually had to threaten legal action in order to get pain relief to the child, who died soon after. To this day I worry that, if her explanatory model was 'right', and mine was 'wrong', what harm might I have done?
> - In the second case (actually this was a very common type of case in Uganda) we were working with an extremely impoverished single mother and her small child who had advanced HIV encephalopathy (brain damage), and who was close to death. Both the mother and the child were poorly nourished. In Uganda healthcare is not free, so patients have to pay for their own medication. In the case of this mother, she was putting literally every shilling she owned into medications which were quite clearly pointless and expensive. We tried to explain to her that she did not need to buy these medications, and that she could stop them. She refused, as she believed strongly that, if she did not do everything she could to prevent the death of loved ones, however apparently futile

that effort may be, her family's ancestral spirits would be aggrieved. The mum continued to buy her drugs, and we provided symptom control, and the child died soon after.

- In the third case (again a common one), we were working with a family of a severely brain-damaged child in the UK. She suffered with prolonged and severe seizures, extremely painful spasms (which were strong enough to dislocate her hips), terrible lung function (due to bad twisted spine and recurrent chest infections), total immobility, very limited communication and almost continuous pain. Her brain damage was such that she could not safely swallow, so she was getting increasingly malnourished and dying. As her body-mass index fell ever further, her specialist GI consultant and her parents decided to admit her to hospital where she was anaesthetised and a feeding tube put in to her stomach. She started to regain weight, but her other symptoms progressively worsened. She started getting abdominal pain and gastric reflux, and she was never free of them for the remaining years of her life. It still troubles me to think that the decision to put in a feeding tube, though it improved her biomedical functioning, only served to prolong her pain and suffering.

In each of these cases, decisions were made that – according to my explanatory models – were not in the 'best interests' of the children concerned. In the first I struggled to cope with the karmic Hindu health beliefs, in the second with the traditional Ugandan health beliefs, and in the third with the biomedical focus on normative standards for planning care and technical intervention. Each model of care I witnessed was an expression of society and culture that I do not feel fully part of, and so perhaps cannot fully understand.

What would your models have led you to think and do if you had been in similar situations?

Activity 3.2: Your explanatory models (30 minutes)

Have a think about what explanatory models you use. Read through the endnotes if you get stuck.

Don't be surprised if you find that you have more than one. Don't even be surprised if you find that the different models that you hold to be 'true' contradict each other.

Remember all self-referential systems end in paradox.

USING EXPLANATORY MODELS SKILFULLY

As we have seen, we understand and interpret our existence from different perspectives. Different perspectives give different understandings, and generate different 'truths'. So while we cannot say with certainty that our existence 'is' anything, we can say that we can view our existence 'as' many things. Health is part of that existence, and any model we use for it will necessarily be partial, limited and subjective.

That is not the same as saying the models are useless, or that they have equal validity. Each model of health has some validity depending on the perspective we take.[20] But there is no one model or approach that is able fully to capture or express the depth and breadth of what it is to be 'healthy' or 'unhealthy'.

As practitioners, we are by definition not theorists. We have to play the hand which we are dealt. When a patient comes to us with a particular health model which differs from our own, we have a number of choices.

- We can use our power advantage to impose our own model.
- We can agree to differ about our health models, and work pragmatically around them.
- We can debate with each other on the relative merits of each and come to an agreement about which to use.
- We can negotiate a compromise 'third model'.

CONFLICTS AND DISSONANCE

Activity 3.3: Patients with different health beliefs (30 minutes)

In this activity I have put in quotation marks some of the words that we imbue, without always realising, with our own subjective beliefs.

Think of the 'kind' of patients that you typically find 'difficult'. You will probably find that there is a 'type' of patient that always seems to get under your skin. Perhaps they are convinced that the 'cause' of their 'problem' is something wholly 'nonsensical' to you; or they have 'strange' ideas about the kind of 'treatment' that might 'work', or they don't seem to be getting 'better' despite the fact you can't find anything really 'wrong'.

Reflect a while on what you 'mean' by all the words in quotes. Are there other 'meanings' for these 'words' that might make 'sense' from a different world-view or explanatory model?

Try to picture an actual patient – one who really makes your heart sink. Allow your mind to settle then allow the patient to come clearly into your consciousness, and visualise an actual situation that you have experienced with this patient.

What sensations do you actually get? Do you feel frustration, disbelief, irritation, or maybe incredulity? Are these sensations pleasant or unpleasant, harmonic or dissonant?

Why does this patient generate these feelings in you?

Over time, and with experience, most of us find our beliefs and models change. In day-to-day practice, however, we rarely have time to consider, reflect and negotiate health beliefs with our patients (although we do a lot subconsciously and almost instantly – *see* workbooks 2 and 4 for more details).

Instead we often come quickly to a tacit and working agreement around those things we need to agree on, and tactfully ignore those things we don't. From patient to patient, we may change position, often subconsciously, in a kind of subtle dance with our patients.

That's not to say consensus is always effective or helpful. Sometimes differences need to be addressed and conflicts brought out into the open air, where they can be analysed and discussed. Conflict can be useful and healthy. It depends a bit on the type of conflict. There are two different types of conflicts that can arise.

- Belief conflicts: for example, a conflict between our beliefs and those of our patients, as in the examples described above. These tend to be a bit easier to deal with, as we don't feel quite so 'invested' in them.

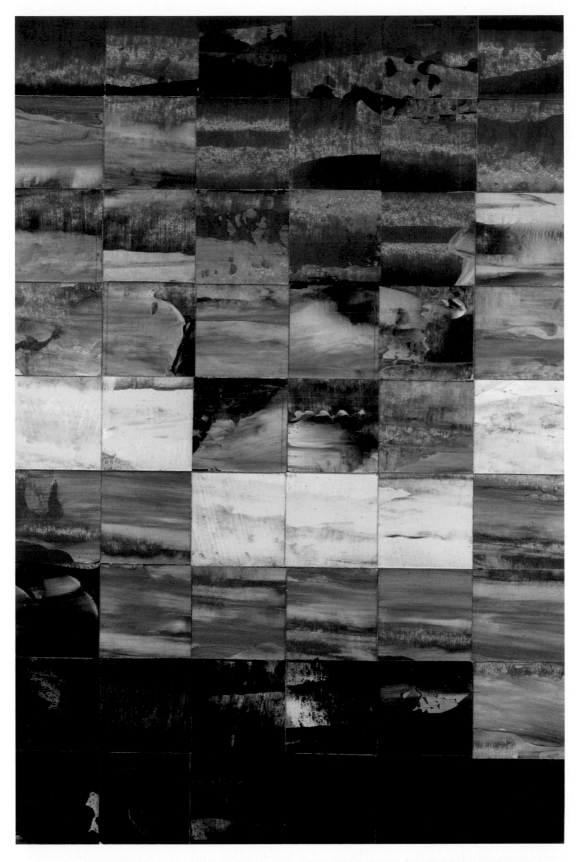

Fractured landscapes like this one by Derek Toon[22] create 'cognitive dissonance', as our minds try desperately to match the fractured reality we are seeing with the ordered and structured beliefs about reality that we hold. But they also ask questions of our consciousness, and particularly ask how much of what we take as 'reality' is in fact many disconnected conscious states glued together by our consciousness.

- Role conflicts: for example, when a patient becomes angry with us (or vice versa), which challenges our self-perceived role as a calm, professional helper who people should like and respect. These tend to be harder to deal with, as they challenge our sense of identity, our sense of who we are.

As health practitioners, we can (and do) get very frustrated and inflamed by these conflicts. But we have another choice. We can see them as opportunities to reflect on, mould and evolve our explanatory models. Health practice is many things, and one of the best things about it is that it is a route for us to find greater awareness, understanding and wisdom.[21]

Ultimately, we may find it useful to remember that models are not realities. Models are always simplistic, otherwise they wouldn't be models – they would be the reality. The reality of existence for our patients and for ourselves may often be far more complex and subtle than any model can capture, which is why we may find ourselves ebbing and flowing from one model into another, often in the same consultation and with the same patient.

INTEGRATING CULTURES AND BELIEFS INTO OUR PRACTICE

As integrated practitioners, we might find it helpful to keep perspective. The messiness of health practice can defy easy modelling. Our existence is highly relational and infinitely complex, and our belief systems may never be able to stretch to meet that infinite complexity.

We therefore might find it helpful to accept dissonance as a fundamental, and very valuable, aspect of our practice. As we practise we will continue to have to mould and change our beliefs as we bump into real-life existence. If we accept this it will be easier to commit and dedicate ourselves to the messy and disordered reality of our existence, recognising that reality in practice always has supremacy over any theoretical models.

We have to act in the 'best interests' of our patients, but that is not to say the patient is always right. There are times when we should challenge and even times we should refuse. But, to give ourselves the best chance of practising 'righteously', we might wish to become aware of our own models, beliefs and prejudices; and to be mindful of these and how they may negatively impact on our patients.

Conflict and dissonance will arise. They are natural and healthy parts of practice. When they do arise, we can choose to ignore them or we can choose to engage with them, communicating both internally with ourselves and externally with our patients, recognising and being thankful for the fact that these moments of dissonance are moments of prime opportunity for our mutual learning and growth.

If we can approach conflicts and dissonance in a humble and open manner, we may find we can find a common understanding that suits both our patients and ourselves. Ideas that seemed off our particular map may begin to make sense when viewed with new eyes. By acting with compassion, and trying to minimise the influence of our pride and vanity, we may find that we can skilfully integrate all of the theories, models and perspectives into one harmonically balanced new co-creation that leads our patients and ourselves to a healthier place.

Much Madness is Divinest Sense

Much Madness is divinest Sense —
To a discerning Eye —
Much Sense — the starkest Madness —
'Tis the Majority
In this, as all, prevail —
Assent — and you are sane —
Demur — you're straightway dangerous —
And handled with a Chain —

— Emily Dickinson[23]

Chapter 4
Information and guidelines

Activity 4.1: Are we experts? (15 minutes)

Next time you are sitting at your desk, or on the ward, or in your consulting room, spend a few minutes reflecting on all the information that is around you.

First, look inside. What information are you aware of? What other information do you 'know' subconsciously? Do you feel like an 'expert'?

Second, look around you. Within your immediate vicinity, how much information do you have access to? Where is it contained? In machines? In books? In people? Do you feel like an 'expert'?

Third, consider all the information there is to know that is 'out there' in the 'noosphere'. Do you feel like an expert?

Finally, think of all the information that is yet to be discovered, if ever.

How do you feel now?

Knowledge is power

– Sir Francis Bacon, *Meditationes Sacræ. De Hæresibus* (1597)

In this chapter we start to come out from within ourselves, and start to look at some of the 'external' tools that we have to master in our practice. Perhaps the most important of these is information.

THE INFORMATION EXPLOSION

The modern world is sometimes defined as the 'information age'. Nowhere is that more true than in the world of health practice.

- As of April 2009, PubMed contained information on 18 782 970 citations in the medical literature and was adding over 670 000 new entries per year.[24]
- The volume of medical literature doubles every 10–15 years.[25]
- In 1989, eight guidelines were published. In 1996 it was 138. Currently there are 7000 medical guidelines published on the Guidelines International Network.[26]

In many ways this explosion of knowledge and its availability is very good. I remember a time when I had to manage my consultations with whatever knowledge was in my head, or in small printed 'handbook' I carried with me. Now I can easily consult my computer or smartphone while I am with my patient and do pretty much everything: look up symptom patterns, find local counselling services, book social services assessments, remind myself of drug doses, email or phone colleagues, arrange ambulances, trigger medical decision support software, or check on the latest football results, all without leaving my desk. But, like all blessings, it can be a curse.

'Information'

This tree has two million and seventy-five thousand leaves. Perhaps I missed a leaf or two but I do feel triumphant at having persisted in counting by hand branch by branch and marked down on paper with pencil each total. Adding them up was a pleasure I could understand; I did something on my own that was not dependent on others, and to count leaves is not less meaningful than to count the stars, as astronomers are always doing. They want the facts to be sure they have them all. It would help them to know whether the world is finite. I discovered one tree that is finite. I must try counting the hairs on my head, and you too. We could swap information.

— David Ignatow[27]

THE EFFECT OF THE INFORMATION EXPLOSION IN PRACTICE

The information explosion has had a significant effect on the way we practise. First, this information revolution has forced us to rethink and redefine our roles.

As we saw in workbook 1, role confusion and role conflict are significant sources of stress in any situation. Traditionally, health practitioners have had a role as 'knowledge experts', acting as a source of information and knowledge. Now patients can access all the knowledge we possess, plus a great deal more. We therefore have to come to terms with the 'expert patient',[28] and that has shifted the power balance between us and our patients.

Which is particularly a problem if we are caught in the God complex . . .

Second, many of us feel that the sheer volume of information is tyrannical at times.

What has become known as 'information overload' is emerging as a significant source of stress for everyone, and particularly for health practitioners. Too much information can result in both poorer decision making and stress. Conversely, too much information can lead us to feel more confident in our decisions than is warranted; presumably because we are not always aware of all the subconscious influences that this information has on our behaviour.

This is not a helpful combination as it leads to stressed health practitioners making poor decisions while at the same time feeling increased confidence and satisfaction with these poor decisions.[29] There is a significant, though elusive, difference between knowledge and understanding.

> Practitioners in the new world should be gatherers of information relevant to individual patient care – the ultimate knowledge broker – instead of hunters preying on the ignorance of their patients to preserve their power and status. The allure of knowledge brokers will be high in a world that suffers increasingly from information overload. Knowledge, we know, is power, but brokering it is more valuable than guarding it.[30]

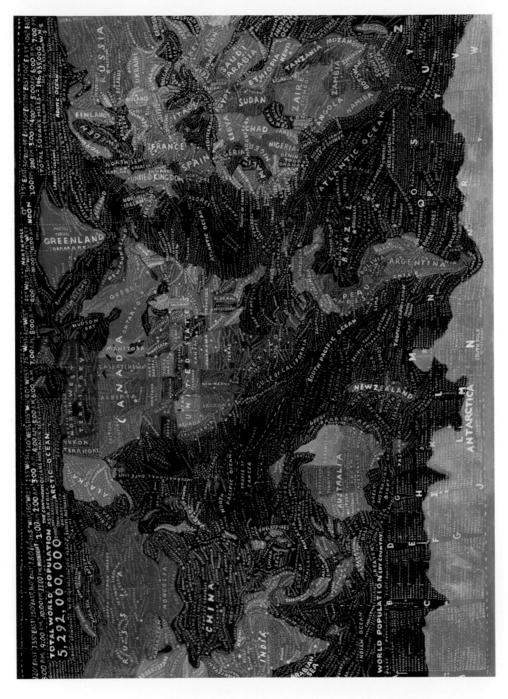

'The World' by Paula Scher is a lovely illustration of how too much information can sometimes make it harder, not easier, to work out where we are trying to go and how we should get there in health practice.[31]

GUIDELINES

Activity 4.2: What 'ought' patients to do (30 minutes)

Have a look at the 'Cate's plot' in the image below, which looks at the risks of heart attacks or strokes in otherwise healthy people given statins. Don't worry too much about the specific statistics. We are looking at the philosophy of 'ought'.

This plot shows visually the results of one particular study, and shows for how many people statins would make no difference (80/100), how many would benefit from statins (5/100) and how many will suffer despite statins (15/100).

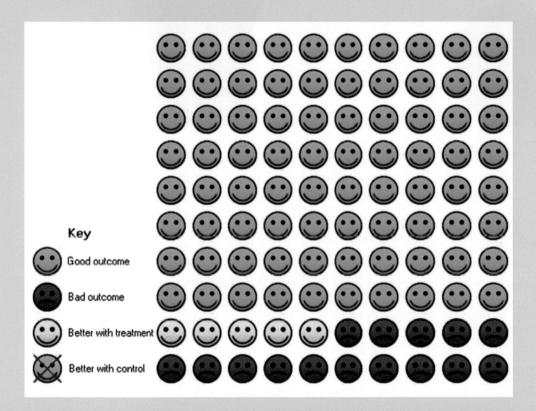

Using these kind of statistics, in the UK we tend to tell patients that they 'ought not' to take statins for primary prevention of vascular disease. But, if we take our practitioner hats off for a second, we can see how subjective this is. For one patient, a 5 in 100 chance of not getting a stroke or heart attack may well seem like a good reason to take statins. For another, a 95 in 100 chance of statins making no difference (either way) would be a good reason not to take them. What patients 'ought' to do does not directly follow logically from empirical evidence.

If you have time, go to Dr Chris Cates' website at www.nntonline.net to look at some other evidence, and even try doing your own.

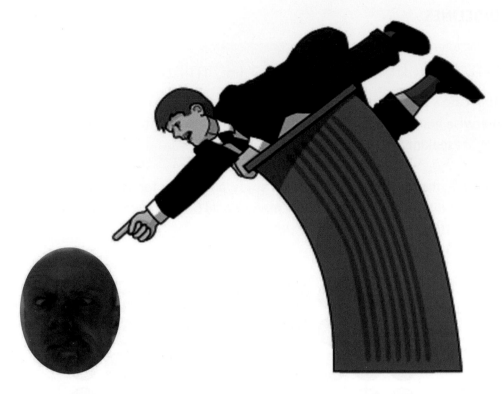

Guidelines and lawyers: when our 'ought' turns against us . . .

While it is already impossible just to assimilate the sheer volume of information that is 'out there', we now also have to cope with an even trickier beast: the guideline. Guidelines are knowledge with 'value added'. They tell us not just what we 'could' do, but also what we 'ought' to do.

But, as we saw in the previous chapters, knowledge claims are also power claims. We live in a world which, in many ways, can be seen as the interplay of different power claims and power struggles.[32] As health practitioners, we try to be apolitical. But that is not the same as being politically naïve. There are many interests at play in health, of which the 'best interest of the patient' is merely one.

Furthermore, as we also saw, moral statements (about what we ought to do) are logically unconnected to empirical statements (about what appears to be the evidence). Therefore, from a philosophical perspective, the validity of guidelines is suspect, and the degree to which practitioners should abide by them is debatable.

This has not stopped many people and groups with many hidden and overt power agendas creating 'guidelines' in order to tell practitioners what we 'ought' to do, even though the guideline writers can have no concept of the specific context of the needs or best interests of the specific patient sitting in front of us. If you are interested in reading a bit of a rant about this, please check out the endnotes![33]

As health practitioners we are often left in a state of heightened anxiety about our lack of knowledge and about our patients, which is only made worse by our apparently justifiable anxiety about our patients' lawyers discovering, exploring and possibly exploiting genuine areas of ignorance about which we have little control.

INTEGRATING INFORMATION AND GUIDELINES INTO OUR PRACTICE

But, let's step back a little, and get some perspective. We cannot stop the growth of knowledge, even if we wanted to. In another 10 years it will be twice as much, in 20 four times, and 30 eight times. Even now, we cannot answer even half of the questions our patients ask us.[34]

As we have seen, knowledge is ultimately infinite and unknowable. But, while we cannot change what is 'out there', we can change what is 'in here' and learn to see knowledge as a tool rather than a tyrant.

Information is an inherent part of existence, and indeed in some respects we quite literally are information, in the form of genetic code. The explosion of accessible information has led to an explosion of knowledge, and that has tremendous potential in health practice.

But as practitioners, we can only know a small fraction of what there is to know, and it is unreasonable for anyone to assume we can know more. Possession of information does not make us expert practitioners, any more than possession of paints makes an expert painter. What makes us experts is how we use the information we have within our grasp to sculpt a healthier, integrated harmonic balance for our patients and ourselves.[35] And if we can help our patients become more expert too, the chance of us sculpting something even more skilful, and even more effective, is greater still.[36]

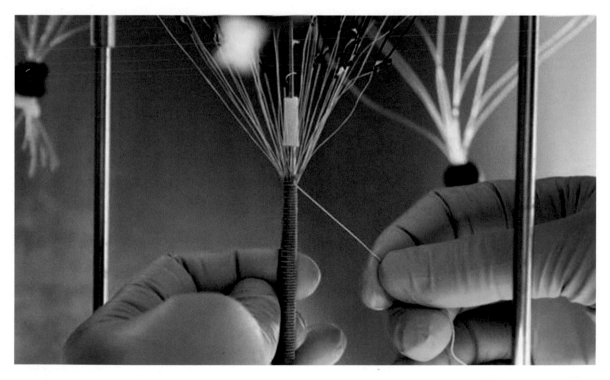

One company (Cytograft Tissue Engineering)[37] is using fine strands of human cellular material to weave coatings for grafts that the patient will then not reject. This is a happy analogy for all health practice. We take our knowledge, the patient's knowledge and 'other' knowledge and weave them into one integrated and balanced whole.

Activity 4.3: Finding 'nothing' at the bottom of 'everything' (30 minutes)

Try this meditation.

Sit comfortably and think of everything there is to know. Now think of everything that you don't know. Imagine all the harm you might have done, be doing, or will do in the future because you don't know everything you could.

Zoom out and become aware of your body. Locate the areas of tension, count your heart rate, feel the speed of your breathing. Let these all begin to drop away, slowing and easing.

As your body relaxes turn your awareness inward, to your thoughts and all the information within you. Visualise these whizzing about chaotically in your mind, or drowning in the glutinous depths of your unconscious. Briefly zoom out again and relax your body.

Come back and this time visualise the thoughts and information as a series of 0's and 1's, like blinking eyes, cheerfully winking at you. Zoom even further out and see yourself as a sculpture, made entirely of minute 0's and 1's, pulsing and winking with life.

Zoom out further and visualise everything around you, your room, your environment, your planet, and the whole universe as a continuous, complex, relational and infinite dance between the 0's and 1's, winking and pulsing against a background of dark nothingness, in a wonderful and breathtaking spectacle.

Spend some time dancing with them, within them, and aware of them.

Gradually come to realise that your practice, your life, your very existence, is your ability to embody, to be aware of and to use that information. You don't have to own it or possess it.

You quite literally are information. Possession of that information does not make you expert. Your expertise is what you do with it: the sculptures you create with it against the infinite background of nothingness.

Chapter 5
Time and resources

We may not agree on everything, but almost all of us would agree that we could seriously use some more time and resources for our practice.

> If only I knew more! If only I had more time! If only I could find funding for that treatment!

Feeling unable to meet the needs of the patient or the moment can leave us feeling conflicted and inadequate.[38]

Activity 5.1: Time and resources (15 minutes)

Run through the last couple of days. Do a little mental audit of the patients you saw. For each one of them, ask yourself:

'Could I have done better if I had more time or resources?'

For how many of them would the answer be 'no'?

Health practice is an expensive business. As health practitioners, wherever we work, we are always up against time, and our resources are always limited. But every contact with a patient has to have a beginning and an end; and there is never enough time or enough resources to address every health concern and every need of any patient.[39]

Managing our resources, our time, and ourselves effectively is therefore a core skill for any health practitioner, and it is skill that requires clear perspective and mindfulness.

THE PROBLEM OF 'FAIRNESS'

Let's get to the heart of it. What we are wrestling with here is 'fairness'. We would like to do more for more people, but we can't. So we have to ration. We ration our time, our money, ourselves.

In time and resource limited settings (and all settings in the universe are time and resource limited) it is natural, and indeed necessary, that we should have debates about the relative effectiveness of different practices, so that we can direct our resources to those that are most effective. That seems only 'fair'.

But fairness is a slippery customer. It is about more than mere equality.[40] We can be unfair even if we treat everyone equally, as some people have higher need than others. Again, choices about whose need is 'higher' depend on what we mean by 'higher', and will also be partly determined by the tool with which we choose to measure. So the ethics of fairness is fraught with subjectivity.

On the other hand, as integrated practitioners we cannot ignore the problem. Without resources, we can do nothing. Even the smallest or simplest health practice requires time and space. Therefore, we are forced to engage, whether we want to or not.

If we have to engage, we may as well try to engage at a skilful, ethical level.

PRACTITIONERS, NOT PRIESTS

As practitioners, we may have particular skills in healthcare that may give our health viewpoints and health claims additional status, but our ethical viewpoints and ethical claims have no particular priority above those of others. Our values and ideas have to compete on a level playing field with those of our patients, colleagues, cultures and societies. Indeed, as we have a vested interest, unless (and even if) we are mindfully self-aware, we may find the moral basis of our opinions may be coloured by self-interest or prejudice, and our decisions distorted by irrationality.[41]

It may be wise to be alive to the possibility that we are not fully aware of ourselves in this matter. We may feel happy to prescribe a cheaper drug, or use a cheaper dressing, or operate from cheaper premises. But are we always happy to move a patient on, when we have done 'enough' for them (even if they don't think we have)? Are we using ourselves effectively and cheaply, or is the way we practise costing a lot in terms of our energy and enthusiasm?

Activity 5.2: Are you prejudiced? (30 minutes)

Our self-interest and prejudice may be more powerful than we care to believe. If you dare, go to the 'Project Implicit' website: https://implicit.harvard.edu/implicit/demo/selecta test.html

Run through the self-tests to discover some unrecognised prejudices. It's quite frightening.

What is even more frightening is that we may have prejudices that we don't think of as prejudices.

For example, we may subtly feel smokers or drinkers should be punished for their actions by receiving a smaller slice of the healthcare pie.

THE BIG (AND SMALL) ISSUES

Health practice is a big issue, but it is not really about 'big issues' like ethics, politics or finance, important though these are. To be effective, we have to focus on what we are skilled at, and do what we do best. We are the kings and queens of the small things. It's what we do, one to one, with each patient, that counts.

As health practitioners, our practice is about dedicating ourselves to trying to help the person in front of us become a little healthier, a little more whole. If we forget that, then we will not fully immerse ourselves in the moment, and we will be less effective as a result.

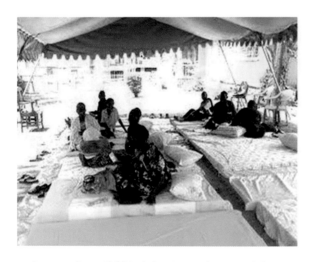 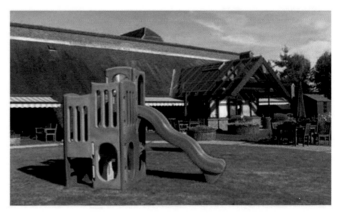

A playground at a children's hospice in the UK and the tent we used to use at the Hospice in Uganda for daycare. Different resource constraints, but it all helped. Whatever resources we have we can use to good effect in creating better health.

And of course, if we have some energy left at the end of our long day, there is nothing to stop us becoming lawyers, politicians or priests too!

PRIORITISING AND CHOOSING

On most days, and in most moments, we are faced with an unachievable multitude of tasks. That mean we need to take perspective. We are humans, not gods (or martyrs).

Once we have this perspective we can try to prioritise what we do, by choosing tasks that most effectively express our values and goals.[42] Prioritisation is a core skill in health practice, and it involves asking ourselves these questions:

- What needs doing?
- Is it my job or could someone else do it more effectively of efficiently?
- If it is my job, is it important?
- If it is important, how urgent is it?

From this chain of thought, and if the job falls best to us rather than someone else, we can rapidly apply an order or priorities:

1   Important and urgent
2   Important but not urgent
3   Urgent but not important
4   Unimportant and not urgent

In practice we tend to get sucked in to the most urgent things, rather than the most important things. But even a moment's thought shows that this is unlikely to be an effective use of our time, energy and money.

Activity 5.3: Prioritise in practice (30 minutes)

Go back to the mental audit you did in Activity 5.1. Think of all the tasks you carried out for your patients, colleagues and organisation. Write them down, in order of 'importance'.

Next to each, write down how much effort or time it took. Is there a clear relationship between the importance of the task and the effort you put in? Be really honest with yourself. It's sometimes hard to accept the possibility that we may be wasting our time and effort.

Reflect on whether there were things you could have said no to, or spent less time on, or delegated to someone more appropriate. How much effort or time would you have saved if you had?

Now think forward. What can and will you do differently?

Visualise yourself completing the important actions. Just as importantly, visualise yourself not completing some of the non-important actions.

Now actually practise doing this in real life. Allow tasks to drop off the end of the list, so that unimportant actions don't get done.

If you feel resistance and internal conflict building in the face of this 'failure', remind yourself you are not God, and you are not perfect. In a constrained universe, it's OK to be constrained. Your constraints allow you to say no, and to fail to do things that are not important. The important thing is that you have succeeded in doing what's most important.

Sometimes, even if it is our job, and even when we have prioritised like this, there are some days when even our 'important and urgent' list is unachievable.

We can become frustrated or upset by this, but it won't help. The list won't get any shorter.

In situations like this, we might wish to remind ourselves of the '80:20' rule[43] (*see* workbook 1, Chapter 5) and decide what actions to take in what order, and what tasks we will leave undone.

It is difficult to overstate the importance of using this technique for rapidly filtering and prioritising tasks. If it is unfamiliar, it is well worth practising, as eventually we can thereby start to automate effective and efficient behaviour.

MINDFUL DEDICATION

Prioritising is not enough. To achieve anything we have to act. But before we act, it is worth inserting a brief pause to become aware and focused.

If we go into the moment conflicted, cross or disempowered by perceived constraints, we will not be fully focused and so less likely to be fully effective. Resource and time constraints are part of our practice, because they are part of existence. We can turn them into tyrants, raging against them or submitting meekly to their power. Or we can choose to focus on our freedom. There are things we can't do, but there are an awful lot of things we can do.

So the first step in starting any task, particularly really urgent and scary ones, is to become mindfully aware. Initially, this means we might wish to become aware of any mind-clutter (such as frustration and anxiety about resource constraints) and then mindfully release that clutter so we can focus single-pointedly on the patient and the moment.

Effective preparation before the moment enables much more effective use of the moment. If, before the consultation starts, we have mindfully read the notes, spoken to relevant people, checked the protocols, rounded up results, addressed any knowledge gaps and briefly brought to mind the patient (if he or she is known), we are more likely to go into the consultation with minds freed up to focus on the patient, and on the moment, and so use time and resources far more efficiently and effectively. If we go in without this clear awareness, everything takes longer and decisions are much less effective.[44]

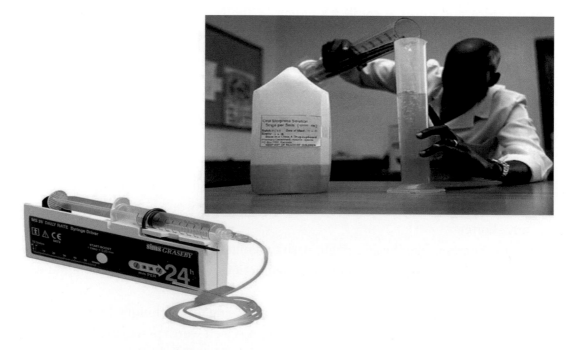

In the UK, we use syringe drivers to give steady doses of pain relief. We didn't have them in Uganda, so Peter would make up our simple oral morphine solution using powder and food colouring. I was surprised to find it worked nearly as well. Both 'worked'.

Activity 5.4: Mindful preparation (30 minutes)

Before your next surgery, or ward round, or clinic, or day at work, consciously insert a few minutes for yourself. If you don't have a second to spare, this may seem like madness. But give it a chance, and see for yourself.

Start by running through a progressive muscle relaxation, or a breathing exercise, or a hypnosis exercise to relax yourself. You don't need to take long. You can do it in a few seconds with a bit of practice.

Now visualise the day ahead: your patients, your colleagues, the likely scenarios. Really try to 'see' yourself in your mind's eye.

Now zoom in. Switch on the rational side of your brain and do a quick problem solve. What's missing? What could you do in advance that would make your day more effective or efficient? What should you avoid doing?

Now zoom out and relax again. Visualise yourself acting effectively and efficiently.

Come back to the present and act how you visualised it.

And smile at yourself when you mess up.

No one is perfect.

BEING FIRM ABOUT WHAT WE CANNOT DO

No practitioner works in isolation. Managing our colleagues, whether bosses, co-workers or juniors, is a core skill for integrated practice. Many people make many demands of us. We can't meet all of them. If someone makes a demand which distracts us from our priorities, we either have to reprioritise, or we have to say no.

Sometimes we have to say no overtly, and sometimes we have to do it covertly, by reducing our availability to others.

- Saying no: because we are not gods, we can't do everything. Different people will have different views about what does need doing. All we can do is try to prioritise according to our purposes and values, and then be honest enough to say no if someone asks us to do something that we do not judge as a high priority (in as compassionate a way as possible). Unless it's the boss . . .
- Minimising interruptions:[45] no matter how good at multitasking we are, being interrupted slows us down because we lose our single-pointed focus. Some interruptions are important, and need priority, but many don't. We can reduce unimportant interruptions by explaining honestly and compassionately to our colleagues how we feel about interruptions, and how we will act when they occur.

Saying no or making ourselves less available sounds easy. But each is very difficult if we are stuck in our complexes. Gods don't do 'weak and fallible' and martyrs can say 'no' to those we feel need us.

In these situations, saying no or making ourselves less available may set up a powerful cognitive dissonance. This internal dissonance may externalise as anger, exasperation or other emotion, which can generate an equal but opposite counter-reaction, and so trigger a negative spiral.

My priorities will rarely be the same as your priorities. So if you ask me to do something which is not on my priority list (and if I am confident that my list will accord with my purposes and values, and that it is prioritised effectively), I have to say no to you.

On the other hand, saying no is not so difficult if we are good enough, honest and compassionate. For that moment, the person requesting assistance becomes the owner of as much attention and empathy as we can spare. If we are going to say no, we can do it in a gentle and honest way. For example:

> 'Look, I can see that you are busy and 'task x' is important to you, but I have an awful lot of other things to do, they are important and urgent, and I am getting tired and need to be gone by five to pick up the kids. I'm sorry I can't help you today.'

Or

> 'Look, this may sound strange, but I am really not good at multitasking and when I get distracted from what I am doing I get forgetful/annoyed/dangerous/panicky. If you need something from me I will be sure to be available to catch up with you at XX.'

Saying no doesn't necessarily mean the task won't get done. We don't work in isolation. Even if a task is not important or for us, very often we work with colleagues for whom it is. So finding that person, and delegating the task to them, is a way of acting effectively with resource and time constraints.

Delegation[46] is not the same as dropping responsibility. When we delegate we maintain a share of responsibility and we also take under our care another person, to whom we have delegated. That means we have to act compassionately, honestly and effectively with them. For example, we might ensure they are ready, capable and supported, give them an opportunity to express concern or say no, and feel safe enough to have a go even if they may make a mistake.

Activity 5.5: Saying no (20 minutes)

Next time you are asked to do something you don't think is important, say no. Do it nicely, but firmly.

It will be scary, so relax and visualise yourself doing it now. Then actually practise it. Visualisation will only take you so far. You may be able to visualise yourself as a brilliant pianist, but it won't make you any good. So stand in front of a mirror and say the words. Feel them rolling out of your mouth, observe your blood pressure going up and your chest clenching. Practise consciously relaxing. Do it over and over until it feels right.

Now take the very next opportunity to do it. Actually say no to a real person. Don't worry if it comes out clumsily to start with. You can always apologise. And we all secretly respect people who have boundaries.

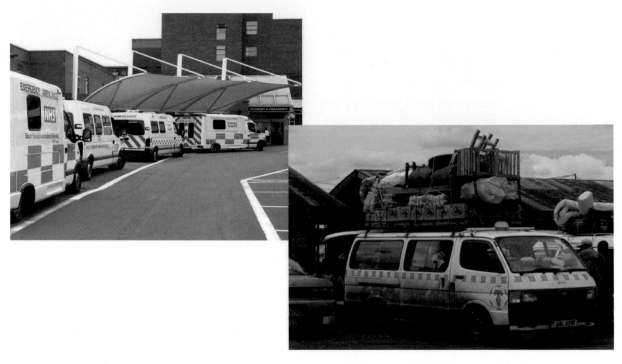

We didn't have ambulances in Uganda. Patients had to squeeze in to the local 'Matatu' buses. It wasn't comfortable, or very safe, but it all worked (after a fashion).

ACTING EFFECTIVELY

Once we are aware of the full context of the situation, clear about our priorities, honest about what is achievable, and mindfully dedicated and single-pointed in our concentration, we can address the task in hand as effectively and efficiently as is possible in that moment. We can then work in relationship with the task in hand to try to create a new and healthier present, whatever that may be.

If that creation is effective, we can feel confident that we have been applying the right skills, and that will boost our confidence and effectiveness next time. If the creation is ineffective, we can check back to make sure it is not because of distraction or other outside factors, and then note that this is a helpful prompt that we have to learn more skills in that area.

Once we have finished acting, we can go back to the beginning of the cycle, becoming aware of a new reality in which we have either succeeded (in which case we can allow ourselves a moment of self-congratulation and maybe an edible or other reward!) or in which we have fallen over but have a new insight into ourselves and the world around us.

This is just to say

This is just to say

I have eaten
the plums
that were in
the icebox

and which
you were probably
saving
for breakfast

Forgive me
they were delicious
so sweet
and so cold

— William Carlos Williams[47]

Chapter 6
Regulations and targets

Activity 6.1: Self-regulation (30 minutes)

Draw two circles.

In the first circle include all the constraints put on you by the regulations of your particular profession. What are you not allowed to do? What would result in you being disciplined? What sort of things are colleagues in your profession disciplined for?

In the second circle, include all the constraints you put on yourself. What standards would you consider were unacceptable to yourself, in terms of how you practise, your probity, the way you present yourself, the expectations you think others should have of you (patients and colleagues). Think more broadly. What would make a 'good-enough' practitioner? What standards would be the lowest you would be prepared to sink to?

Now zoom out and compare the two circles. Which is bigger? Which contains more? Which set of standards is more exacting?

Regulations and targets can be tools or tyrants, depending on what perspective we take. We are dealing with people who are ill and vulnerable, so trust and respect are important to us. Without them we would be less effective. So we don't want to get tarred by the same brush as unskilful, ill-informed, lazy or dishonest colleagues, who might harm patients. It is helpful for us to have systems to identify, correct or exclude people like this in our professions.

In my working lifetime in the UK we have had some pretty dreadful cases of health practitioners stepping right out of reality into major God-complex mode, harming and killing patients en route (for example, Beverly Allot, and Harold Shipman); failing even on basic levels to care for vulnerable children (Victoria Climbie and Baby P); harming patients with poorly tested drugs (e.g. thalidomide); and of course many other cases where practitioners have deliberately misled and defrauded patients when they are at their most vulnerable.

On the other hand, sometimes we can feel oppressed, inhibited or even frightened by these regulations and targets.

Most regulations in health practice dictate that we should be technically competent, keep up to date, maintain reasonable and non-coercive relationships with patients and colleagues, do our bit in teaching and training students and junior colleagues, and behave in an honest and upstanding fashion. The standards set by these rules and regulations are usually quite low, as they represent the 'bottom line' below which we should not fall. Therefore, most of us, most of the time, steer well clear of crossing their boundaries. For example, the number of doctors in the UK struck off per year is around only 0.02% of the total, and fewer than 0.005% are struck off for clinical incompetence.[48] Most are struck off for inappropriate relationships, dishonesty, drug and alcohol abuse, or indecency.

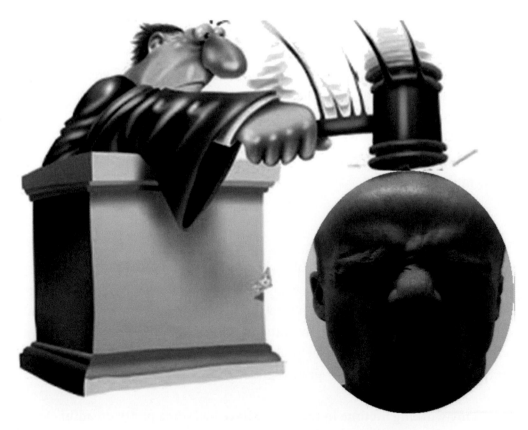

Regulations – they give us all a headache, but perhaps more anxiety than is necessary?

In other words, while we might worry about regulations and licensing issues, the actual evidence suggests we have very little to fear as long as we are honest and decent. Perhaps we can even look at regulations as useful tools, protecting both patients and practitioners against poor standards, fraud, abuse and quackery, and protecting the standing and trustworthiness of our professions.

TARGETS

At the other end of the scale from regulations are targets. Most of us have some targets to reach as part of our contracts with our employers, clients or governments.

Sometimes, targets can be helpful tools. When tied to evidence of effectiveness, they may help us to focus our efforts on the most useful and 'effective' practices (*see* Chapter 9), and waste fewer resources in ineffective practices. They may also encourage us to remember to focus on things that are important, but about which the patients may not be aware (for example, health screening, disease prevention and health promotion).

Sometimes, however, targets can be tyrants: *'When a measure becomes a target, it ceases to be a measure.'*

In the UK at the moment, we are working in a target-based culture within which a large proportion of our income is related to achievement of targets. Whenever I sit down at my desk to consult, my computer constantly generates a stream of pop-up boxes telling me what to examine, what tests to do,

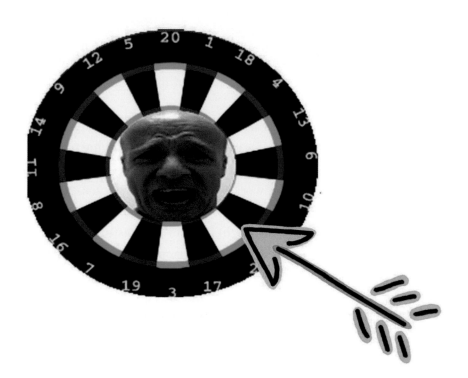

We may feel that we can never escape targets, but we can use them more or less skilfully.

what drugs to prescribe (and not prescribe) and what screening needs to be done. I have just carried out an informal survey in my own practice and found I average nine 'messages' per consultation, telling me what to do and what not to do. What's more, at the end of surgery I will go through my emails and read about audits I need to prepare and reports I need to write in order to meet our contractual obligations as a practice.

Activity 6.2: Targets (20 minutes)

Take a deep breath. List down every single target that you are expected to achieve by your government, your profession, your organisation, your team, your boss or anyone else.

Take another deep breath.

Let's try to be even-handed here.

Next to each of these targets make a note of how effective that target has been in improving the effectiveness of the care you (or your colleagues) provides. Perhaps score it or just write something like 'not very', 'quite' or 'very'.

What proportion of the targets you have listed have you categorised as being useful?

Reflect on that for a while. Is it worth 'saying no' to any of them?

Targets can be useful tools in health practice. In many countries, governments and health organisations appear to have reduced illness and mortality in a range of different conditions.[49]

On the other hand, sometimes targets can be tyrants. Targets are always forms of disguised 'power claims', with various interest groups trying to set the agenda, often under the cloak of an 'evidence base'. Where the interests of the patients overlap with the vested interest, they can work well. Where they don't, targets can undermine good healthcare. They may cause us to lose our focus on the specific experience and problems of the individual patient in front of us, waste time on targets that do not improve the health of the individual, or discriminate against patients with conditions other than those targeted. Financially incentivised targets may set up a conflict of interest for the practitioner, as we may be forced into choosing between what is in the best interest of the patient and what is in our own financial interest.[50]

This is an interesting graph showing the effects of financial incentivisation of family doctors in the UK by the National Health Service. It shows both the strengths

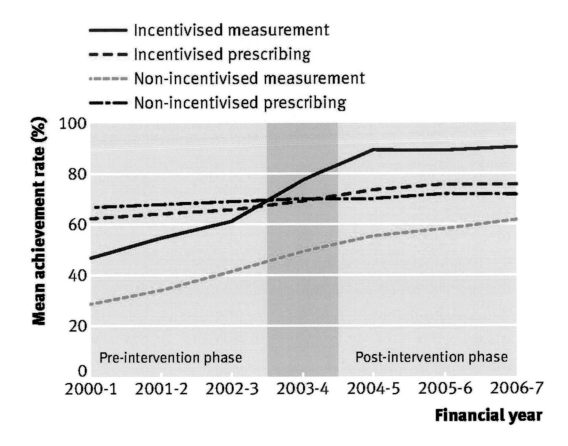

Effect of incentivised health targets in the UK[51]

and weaknesses of targets. Targeted areas improve more than background trend, but non-incentivised target areas improve less than background trend.[52] So, in this case, targets lead to both better health and worse health.

INTEGRATING REGULATIONS AND TARGETS INTO OUR PRACTICE

Regulations and targets are always there, as an 'other', at the back of our minds, and we are aware of the stories of colleagues who have fallen foul of them. Like the terrible bedtime stories of our childhood, these sorry tales have the ability to keep us awake at night, particularly at times we are struggling. In that regard, heavy-handed regulation and targets can act as tyrants, undermining and distorting our confidence and our practice.

However, we can take some perspective. Regulations can be tools, in that they enable our patients to trust us and ensure that we and our colleagues practise at least at a reasonable standard. Because of these standards and this trust, we get paid to do jobs that are rewarding and respected. Targets can help us to focus on areas that may slip our minds, or be priorities for particular groups or organisations. We all play *in* teams, so it may be wiser where possible to play *as* a team.

There may be times where we fall foul of targets or regulations. But if we commit ourselves to values that are compassionate, and lead professional lives that are honest and fair, and if we avoid taking advantage of our patients, the chance of us being seriously disciplined is vanishingly small.

When we can attain and hold this perspective, regulations and targets stop being shackles, holding us back. If we can accept we are good enough, they can become useful tools that we can use, or not, as we explore the far broader and deeper oceans of our practice and existence.

You took away all the oceans

You took away all the oceans and all the room.

You gave me my shoe-size in earth with bars around it.

Where did it get you?

Nowhere.

You left me my lips, and they shape words, even in silence.

– Osip Mandelstam[53]

Chapter 7

Organisations and teams

Activity 7.1: Your organisation (30 minutes)

Spend some time considering the organisation within which you work.

Note down its strengths. How does it make your work more effective, more efficient or more enjoyable? How do you help it function more effectively and efficiently? Note these down too.

Note down its weaknesses. How does it hinder your effectiveness, efficiency or enjoyment? Now turn the tables. Are there any ways you hinder its efficiency or effectiveness?

Zoom out. On balance, does your organisation act as a tool or as a tyrant to your health practice?

Sometimes, we love being at work. There are few things more rewarding than feeling part of a good team, pursuing shared values and goals, in an effective and constructive way.

Other times, going to work feels like stepping into Hades. It seems to suck the life, enjoyment and hope right out of us.

As practitioners, almost all of us work in organisations, however small. These days it is very difficult for us to meet even the basic requirement of offering safe and effective healthcare without adequate teams and organisations around us and supporting us. But, within our organisations, we hope to do 'well'. Doing well may be about money and acclaim, and indeed these are important.

Few of us can honestly say we would work for free.

However, we may also work because work gives us the opportunity to create and express an existence that reflects our values and our beliefs about what is important in life. In that way, we look to our organisation to give us the support and the opportunity to grow and to express ourselves ever more expertly, as we develop in skill and experience.

ORGANISATIONS AS TOOLS AND TYRANTS

Organisations can be both tools and tyrants. Like persons, they are highly complex, relational entities, because they are made up of people, working with other people, for other people within a framework of targets, objectives, finance, laws, regulations, environment and politics.

Also like persons, organisations can have 'personalities', although we tend to use the term 'organisational culture' instead. Organisational cultures change constantly in response to influences from within and without the organisation.[54] Like people, organisations are created, can thrive and evolve, or weaken and die. Organisations and teams are, in many ways, extensions of ourselves, in that we express ourselves through them, and they express themselves through us.

Through our organisations, we also learn and utilise our interdependence on others, and we have an opportunity to practise compassion by providing support for them to grow and express themselves as well.

As individuals within organisations, we therefore have responsibility to care compassionately, honestly and in a balanced way for our colleagues, our teams and our organisations. In the same way, our colleagues, teams and organisations have responsibility to care compassionately, honestly and in a balanced way for us. There is a balance to be struck between our personal needs and the needs of the organisation.

Neither should become sick at the hand of the other.

MOTIVATION

We are more effective if we are motivated.[55] As we saw in workbook 1, Maslow suggested that we have a hierarchy of needs, ending in the full actualisation of ourselves. Herzberg suggested that our organisations are able to provide us with the opportunity for self-actualisation, and suggested certain factors that may demotivate us, and factors that may motivate us.

We may become demotivated if we do not have clear roles or objectives, good working relationships, a reasonable minimum salary, and a safe and reasonably pleasant working environment. It also appears that we may become more motivated by a sense of achievement, recognition for our work, a sense of challenge, work we find interesting, and opportunities for growth, learning and development.

Activity 7.2: Your job satisfaction (20 minutes)

Try this job satisfaction inventory (from Open Door Coaching*) to reflect on how satisfied you are at work. To determine your score, total of all numbers you have circled. The highest possible score is 51 and the lowest is 17. Scoring: 40–51 High level of satisfaction, 27–39 Medium level of satisfaction, < 27 Low level of satisfaction.

I like my current job.	1	2	3
I am clear about my career direction and life purpose.	1	2	3
It is easy for me to set goals for myself.	1	2	3
I usually attain the goals I set.	1	2	3
I have no fears about changing jobs.	1	2	3
I think of myself as a successful person.	1	2	3
I have high self-esteem.	1	2	3
Once I decide to make a change in my life, I usually move ahead and do so without making excuses or procrastinating.	1	2	3
I view change as a healthy occurrence.	1	2	3
The work environment in my current job meets all of my needs.	1	2	3
I know exactly which career field I want to enter (or in which I want to stay).	1	2	3
I understand what motivates me to work, and I make job choices based on those factors.	1	2	3
I understand the inner needs that I feel a job should fulfil.	1	2	3
My inner needs are fulfilled through my work.	1	2	3
I know the signs that tell me when it is time for me to change jobs or careers.	1	2	3
I enjoy nearly all of the tasks performed in my job.	1	2	3
My job allows me to satisfy my personal values and fulfil my personal goals as I do the work.	1	2	3

Source: Open Door Coaching. *Job satisfaction inventory.*[56]

THE FUNCTIONS OF HEALTH ORGANISATIONS

Organisations have varied functions.[57] If the organisation is to be efficient and effective, we hope these functions work together in an integrated, harmonically balanced way.

As health practitioners the team and organisation around us are very important, as they provide very important facilitating and holding functions.[58] We deal with people who are suffering, and we are paid by our societies both to relieve and to contain that suffering. Relieving suffering is a complex task, requiring more skills and resources than any one person can provide. Containing suffering is not easy. So, as we saw in workbook 1, our work can occasionally make us stressed, burnt out or unwell.

Without organisations and teams around us, we are less able to relieve or contain suffering effectively, less able to function effectively, and without people to support and cover for us when we are struggling or need a break.

To be efficient and effective, the people, functions and resources within an organisation hope to work together in an integrated, harmonically balanced way. That means the effective organisation looks for the following.

- Clarity of purpose: for each individual and for the whole organisation.
- Provision of sufficient resources, time and leadership for the people who work within it to achieve their goals.
- Systems for training, supervising, monitoring and evaluating people and processes.
- Good communication systems both with and without.

DYSFUNCTIONAL ORGANISATIONS

Poorly run organisations and poor leadership are a significant source of stress for health practitioners.[59] Work overload, a sense of loss of control, unclear home–work boundaries, resource constraints, fear of job loss, poor discipline, bullying or other abuse, too much change and unrealistic goals all reduce our resilience and make us more liable to unhelpful stress and eventual burnout. Sadly, these entities are all too common in healthcare organisations.

When we work in poorly managed organisations, it begins to have negative effects not just on us as individuals but also on our teams. Integrated practitioners do not become immune to suffering and loss because we remain compassionate. The cost of that compassion is that we endure some of our patients' suffering and loss too. We therefore hope that our colleagues and organisations will continue to support and hold us, so we can maintain our professionalism in the face of suffering and loss. If they cannot, the suffering can become turned within, tyrannising individuals, groups and even whole organisations.

> As part of my work in family practice and palliative care, both in the UK and abroad, I have worked with a lot of teams that are under stress or failing. Whether in family practice or children's palliative care, whether in

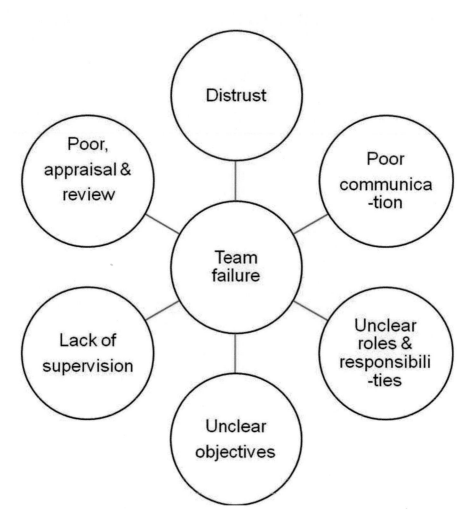

Some causes of team failure

UK or Africa, my experience of team failure is that it is usually due to poor management, or lack of resources, or both. In trying to help these teams and organisations back onto their feet, I have become ever more aware of the importance of our immediate teams in health practice. With good, supportive, open and tolerant teams, it is amazing how much individuals are able to hold and manage. If teams are dysfunctional, everything and everyone suffers.

When a team becomes unable to contain and hold its members, either because the degree of suffering is too great for it to manage or because there are problems with team cohesion, the team can begin to 'split'. Splitting may manifest in various ways. Sometimes bullying emerges, with some members picked on and used as scapegoats for expression of the pain. At other times the team may split into cliques, with cliques expressing the pain as inter-group conflict. Or the team may 'go slow', becoming avoidant to change or creativity. Or the team as a whole may become sick, gradually losing healthy members to other organisations and unhealthy members to sickness.

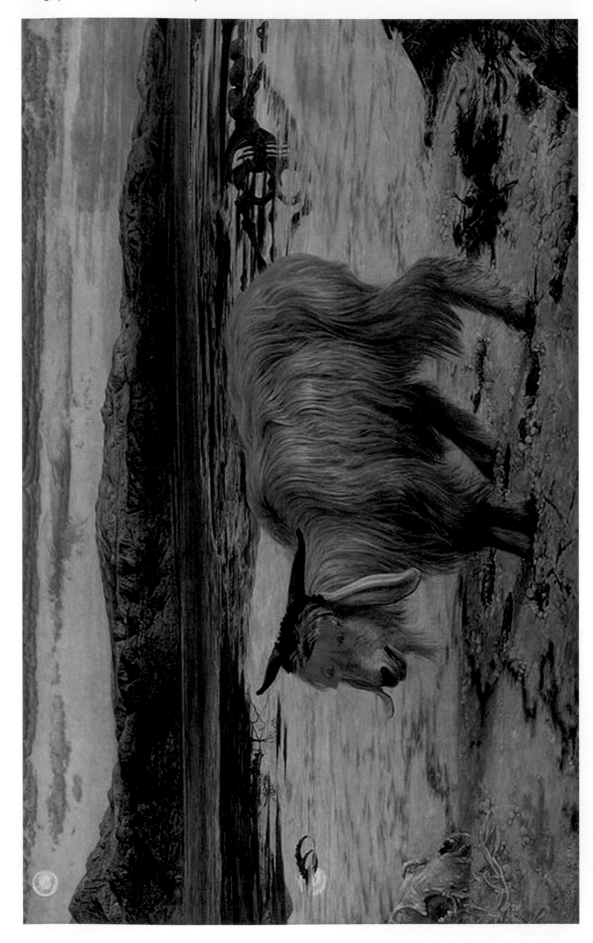

The Scapegoat – with apologies to Holman Hunt

ASSESSING OUR ORGANISATIONS

In the same way we can assess, diagnose and manage our patients, we can also assess, diagnose and manage our organisations.

There are now numerous ways we can do this, using tools that have been developed for many organisations in many fields. The kind of information generated by these tools is useful both to ourselves (if we can see something is wrong we will identify less strongly with the troubles) and also to our bosses (who may also be feeling out of their depth and for whom it may provide concrete and useful information with which to work).

There are many pre-prepared tools that we can use for this purpose, and they are itemised in the endnotes.[60] For example, we can assess our

- team functioning: using Belbin Team Roles, or Myers-Briggs Team Inventory
- performance appraisal and management: using audits, significant events, and clinical supervision tools
- relationship with our patients: using patient satisfaction tools
- teaching and training tools: using learning styles and learning needs tools
- organisational responsibility and ethical action assessments
- analysis of the effectiveness of processes for organisational decision making and problem solving
- assessment of staff motivation
- management and assessment of tolerance to change.

Have a look through some of them, and try them out. Or use the brief organisation appraisal tool in Activity 7.3.

Activity 7.3: Appraise your organisation (30 minutes)

Ask yourself these questions about your organisation and note down the answers

- Are we clear about the values of our team and organisation?
- Are we clear about the objectives of our team and organisation?
- Do we all have clear job and role descriptions?
- Are these accurate, fair and manageable?
- Is there a culture within which we can learn together and learn from our mistakes together?
- Is there tolerance within our organisation for the natural peaks and troughs of health practice?
- Do we get a chance for appraisal, where we can review time past, reflect on the present and make plans for the future?
- Does our team get sufficient and effective time for discussion, reflection, offloading and supporting each other?
- Have you avoided any signs of team dysfunction, such as bullying, scapegoating, clique formation or change avoidance?
- When we manage difficult cases, get upset, or make mistakes, do we have the opportunity to debrief and learn with each other?

If the answer to any of these is no, then communication may be partly blocked. Poor communication leads to poor team-working and poor morale, and poor team-working and poor morale leads to poor patient care.

What can you do to improve this?

HOW CAN WE HELP OUR ORGANISATIONS WORK MORE EFFECTIVELY?

There is a wealth of literature now available about coaching, supervision, training, and change management; some of the more useful ones can be found in the endnotes.[61] However, there are five elements that seem to be crucial for health practitioners working within teams and organisations. These are as follows.

Ensure you have a clear and accurate job description and personal objectives with proper review

If we don't know what is expected of us we will flounder, our boundaries won't be clear, we will keep making the same mistakes over and over and we will miss opportunities to develop. Clear job descriptions, clear knowledge of our objectives, formal feedback from colleagues and a regular appraisal or review all help us to survive and thrive.

Ensure you have adequate supervision

Feeling out of our depth or unsure of our direction is frightening and unsettling. Health practice is stressful enough without having to deal with that as well. Regular supervision, one to one or as a team, provides a system for talking through difficult cases or mistakes, sharing problems, sifting solutions and planning the way forward.

Ensure you have team support

We all struggle from time to time, whereas at other times the lights are all green and we seem to fly through. If we can meet regularly with colleagues, the chances are different members will be at different stages of the cycle, and those who are flying can support those who are struggling. What goes around comes around, and soon the team will develop a sense of group responsibility and trust for each other. If we notice bullying, scapegoating, clique formation or change avoidance building in our team, we have responsibility for trying to address it by raising it with our peers or managers, and to help our organisations become more balanced, compassionate and effective.

Set yourself good boundaries

We need opportunities and time for breaks, support, supervision and training. 'Stay late' syndrome may be a sign of God or Martyr complexes. To function effectively over the long term, we can ensure that the demands placed on us are within our capacity, and that we have built in some tolerance for the natural peaks and troughs of health practice. If our work demands are outside our control, it is not ideal to put up with it, as we will end up harming our teams, our patients and ourselves.

Be gentle and realistic

Just as we cannot be perfect, nor can our teams and organisations.

We spend a lot of time together with colleagues and so it is not unusual for our organisations and teams to generate strong emotions. Sometimes these emotions are positive, but sometimes not. When considering this mindfully, we may be surprised at how strong our attachments are, and how powerfully our organisations, teams and colleagues can affect the way we feel and the way we think.

It is important to recognise the difference between dedication and attachment. We can be dedicated to our team and colleagues, but we are not identified with them. If our organisation is weak, it doesn't mean we are. If we expect our organisation or team to be perfect, should we expect ourselves to be perfect too? Just as we only need to be good enough, so our organisations only need to be good enough.

But if we are faced with a situation where we do not believe in the values or practices that we are being asked to share and to express, we have a responsibility to enter a dialogue with our organisation in an attempt to realign our values, the organisation's values, or both. If we cannot align, we have a responsibility to ourselves to make a choice about whether to change organisations or stay and cope with the misalignment. But it is not compassionate, honest or effective, either for us or the organisation, to stay and become demotivated and possibly unwell.

> It may be that you are in a dysfunctional organisation, and despite all your best efforts, that dysfunction seems too deeply rooted for you to correct. If so, you have a stark choice, but a clear one. Do you want to allow your health to be sucked away by the darkness at the heart of your organisation? If not, walk away.

INTEGRATING ORGANISATIONS AND TEAMS

At their best, organisations and teams give us the opportunity to quite literally merge consciousness with other individuals to co-create a new existence, and one that is better than the one before. In working together we can achieve so much more than in working alone. We are social animals, islands of relationality designed to fit snugly into ever more complex levels of relationality. So working together is not just a job, it is a natural expression of our existence, within which we are able to create something truly special, definitely intangible, and perhaps even miraculous – the better health of our patients, of each other and of our organisations, all at the same time.

Just as cells within an organism, we each have our role and task, and when we can each fulfil them the whole organisation will work more effectively. We each therefore have a responsibility to do our job and to identify and correct dysfunction.

But unlike cells in an organism, we can survive independently. We always have the option to walk into work, and to walk out again. Our creation is in our own hands. So we have a responsibility to that too.

Working Together

We shape our self
to fit this world

and by the world
are shaped again.

The visible
and the invisible

working together
in common cause,

to produce
the miraculous.

I am thinking of the way
the intangible air

passed at speed
round a shaped wing

easily
holds our weight.

So may we, in this life
trust

to those elements
we have yet to see

or imagine,
and look for the true

shape of our own self,
by forming it well

to the great
intangibles about us

— David Whyte[62]

Chapter 8

Space and the environment

Activity 8.1: Your space (30 minutes)

Walk into the space that you usually practice in, as if for the first time. Apply the mindfulness techniques discussed in workbook 1 to allow your muscles to relax, your adrenaline to drain away and your mind to clear. Systematically use your five senses:

What do you see around you? Look and try to see all the details.

Close your eyes and open your ears. Listen for the loud sounds, then the quieter ones, and then for the silences too.

Refocus on your body. What can you feel?

Finally, open up your senses of smell and taste. Try to extricate each individual taste and smell, naming them if possible, or giving them form or colour if not.

Now come back to yourself. What is the space saying to your mind? How does it make you feel?

Would you say it is a therapeutic space? Does it make you feel healthier?

Unlike actors and artists, health practitioners may not be as aware of the importance of space or of how we use it within our practice. But we are, at one level, both artists and actors. Therefore, we can use space more or less skilfully.

A well-loved space radiates that love.

— Diana Lalor[63]

WHAT DOES OUR SPACE SAY?

We have all had experience of how the space and environment around us can affect how we feel. In trying to become more skilful practitioners, the ability to manipulate the space around us is an essential but sadly rather underused one.

In thinking about how to set up our practising space, it is helpful to think of what we might wish the space to 'do', and also what we wish the space to 'say'.

This might seem like a strange concept, but we are able to develop relationships with space, in the same way we can develop relationships with people. There are some spaces with which we feel safe and familiar, and others with which we feel unsafe and unfamiliar.[64] We usually want our patients to feel secure and comfortable with us, so it makes sense to try to ensure that they feel secure and comfortable in our space.

CHANGES IN HEALTH PRACTICE SPACE

It may not be something that we are aware of, but the 'space' of Western health practice has changed dramatically in the last century.[65] Prior to that, health practice was largely carried out in the home, and was therefore integrally bound up with people, families, culture and society.

As 'disease' has become extracted both from the home and (in some ways) from the person, so the space in which we practise health has also changed. Health has become more technical, fragmented and specialised, and our health practice environment has done likewise. For most of us, the space in which we now practise has become quite divorced from the home, in look, feel and experience.

Perhaps, in our search for ever greater understanding of the story and the expression of illness and disease, we have become ever more divorced from the reality of the personal experience of them. To get an idea on how much things have changed, in a relatively very short time, read this description of a family practice in the UK in the 1930s.

> The surgery was a room leading off from the doctor's smoking room. The walls were distempered in dirty, dark red. The floor was of bare boards and the room ill-lit by a small gas jet from his own plant. It contained a desk which was rarely used, and half a dozen chairs. There was no examination couch and no washbasin.
>
> The old patients adored him and gladly waited for hours – half a day or longer if necessary. They sat in a stone bench around the pump in the yard if the weather was fine, or on the chairs in the surgery (with the doctor) if wet.[67]

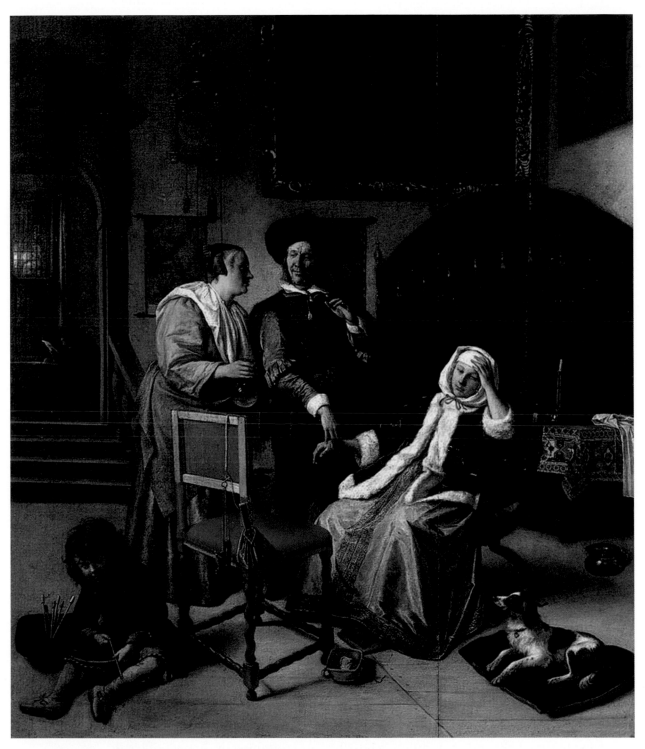

'Doctor's Visit' – by Jan Steen[66]

THERAPEUTIC ENVIRONMENTS

Of course there are many good reasons why we can't go back to practising in 'distempered rooms' or leaving our patients outside (much as we may sometimes wish to!) Indeed, we may have very limited scope for changing our environments. Environments are dictated by their function, by the technology they house, by rules and regulations, by cost, and by many other factors. Nevertheless, there are some things we can do to shape and sculpt our space, and so make it more integrated and harmonically balanced with our practice and with our lives.

Space that is integrated like this can be said to be more 'therapeutic' because it gives us a sense of belonging, safety, containment and empowerment.[68]

How people relate to their space seems to be culturally conditioned.[69] The way we 'fix' our space with walls and boundaries; the way we subdivide our space with furnishings and plants; the way we use the individual space around our bodies: all if these vary from culture to culture.[70]

As practitioners, we usually care for people from many different and diverse cultures and subcultures. So the more flexibly we sculpt our space, and the more care we take in not making our space too closely tied to one culture or another, the more likely our patients will feel safe, contained, empowered and informed and also feel they belong.

MAKING CONSULTING SPACE MORE THERAPEUTIC

As all these things are culturally conditioned, it is not possible to write here for all cultures, even if I were able to do so. So we will just stick to suggestions for 'Western' settings, in the hope that these might be of interest to practitioners in other settings, and help them think through their own cultural factors in their own space.

If we work primarily from consulting rooms, things that might sculpt our space to make it safer and more comfortable would include the following.[71]

- Including some 'personal' touches to reduce the clinical atmosphere, but taking care not to overdo it. It is important to make the space neutral enough so that patients feel they belong there too.
- Not letting our space 'shout' at our patients (for example, by putting lots of 'educational' posters and images around which may hector and scare them).
- Reducing clutter (interestingly, clutter seems to make people more aggressive, less focused and even more prejudiced in their thoughts and behaviour[72]).
- Screening off or hiding away possibly offensive equipment.
- Using fragrances to counter clinical smells.
- Using natural light and air as much as possible, and softening the impact of harsh overhead lighting where possible.
- Allowing sufficient space so that there is no sense of intrusion on the patient's personal space (for example, by leaving seats unfixed so that people can move them to suit their preference).

- Making a clearly defined boundary between the 'public areas' and the semi-private area of the waiting space, using strategic placing of furniture and plants.
- Organising our consulting space so that it encourages easy communication (for example, removing physical barriers between the patient and practitioner).
- Giving some control to the patient (for example, chairs that can be moved or cushions that can be held in a lap).
- Using colours and forms that positively affect mood and security (for example, soft, curving and circular forms, pastel colours or creams, blues and greens).
- Using textures that comfort or calm or stimulate touch.

Activity 8.2: What do we teach about practice space? (15 minutes)

I found this 'brief checklist' in an article from a medical journal explaining to GP trainees the key factors they should consider when setting up their consulting rooms.

- A comfortable working environment.
- A good stock of equipment at all times.
- Access to learning resources during and between consultations.
- Access to good-quality patient leaflets.
- An in/out tray to ease paperwork pressures.

What is missing?
Write another list, for yourself.

MAKING HOSPITAL ENVIRONMENTS MORE THERAPEUTIC

In Western 'conventional' health practice we read and teach very little about how we should use our space as a tool to improve our patients' and our own health, but there is evidence that it makes a real and quantifiable difference, including:[73]

- reduced staff stress and fatigue
- reduced risk of infectious diseases
- reduced risk of injury
- reduced medication errors
- reduced psychological distress and depression
- reduced confusion in elderly patients
- greater effectiveness in delivering care
- improved patient safety
- improved health outcomes
- improved overall healthcare quality.

There are many therapeutic factors over which we as individual practitioners have no control and cannot change, because they are already designed and built into (or

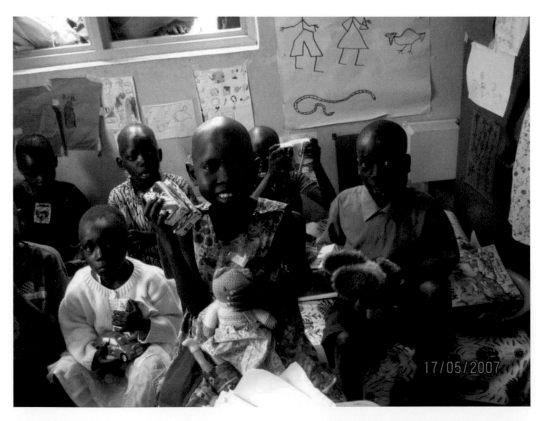

In the children's cancer ward at Mulago Hospital in Kampala we worked with the local team and volunteers to set aside some space for children which we painted then decorated with their own paintings and some toys. One of the doctors on the ward was delighted by the result. 'They have just emerged from under their blankets for the first time,' he said.

out of) the building. These might include things like good ventilation, good lighting, entry of natural light, noise reduction and so on.

Nevertheless, there are some small things that we can do to make a difference, for example:

- keeping noise down, particularly during sleep times
- allowing domestic objects such as pictures, ornaments and cushions on to the ward
- improving patient orientation through clearer signage, better information and explanation
- enabling patients to access bright light (preferably natural light) as much as possible
- using distractions such as music, companion animals and laughter
- using art (particularly representational art, as abstract art seems to generate quite powerful negative reactions in some people)
- providing access to nature, either real (if gardens and balconies are possible) or represented through pictures
- making small changes (where possible) to the general layout, colour scheme, furniture, floor covering, curtains and so on (*see* the section on consulting rooms above).

INTEGRATING OUR SPACE INTO OUR PRACTICE

Ultimately, the most important factors in our practice space are the patients and us.

This is a rather strange concept, but science suggests that space and time are relational entities that we can only (and always) experience through the medium of our consciousness. In other words, time and space have no 'meaning' except as conceptual representations.[74]

This concept can be hard to grasp, particularly if we have been brought up to see ourselves as objective 'observers' of a concrete 'reality'. But a moment's thought shows it to be true. We 'perceive' energy, matter and forces from the universe around us and within us. From these perceptions our consciousness creates the world that we experience, and which is so much richer than simply energy, matter and force. In other words we create our existence, in a continuous interplay with perception, as we go along.

As our consciousness is self-created, so we quite literally create our own experience of space. When we are in relationship with other conscious beings (like patients) that creation is shared. Therefore, in relationship with our patients we quite literally co-create our experiences of the space we operate within.

In practice, what this means is that we can influence how we and our patients experience our space. But in order to do that we might wish to become aware of our own subconscious influences on it.

To get perspective, we can look at ourselves and our practice space as if for the first time, or as if we have just stepped off a spaceship from a different planet. Or

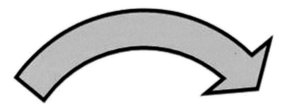

Perception   Creation

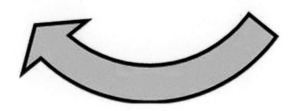

we can imagine ourselves as one of our patients: a child maybe, or someone with disabilities, or someone from a culture wholly different to our own. We can sit on the floor, or stand on a chair, to try to see it from unusual angles and lights.

We can also think about what we are trying to achieve through our healthcare practice and then ask ourselves: 'How does the space that we occupy help or hinder me from achieving those values and goals?'

Activity 8.3: Sculpting your space (30 minutes)

Sit down in front of a mirror looking at yourself in your place of work, and preferably from the perspective and position your patients normally take. If you can't actually do it, do it in the mirror of your mind. Relax and allow your minds to clear, and gradually notice things you have not noticed before. Emotions will emerge and disperse as your attention mindfully focuses on different elements of what you see. Are these positive or negative emotions?

Now reflect on what your body and environment are saying. Are they saying what you want them to say? Do the messages concur with your values and goals? Is there enough of 'you' in the space? Or maybe there is too much of 'you' in the space? Will your patients feel that they belong, and that they are safe, contained, informed and enabled in your space?

Now it is time to act to sculpt your space. Change what you can, and be at peace with what you can't. Most importantly, in your space, remember to create and sculpt some space for yourself. Just something small is enough. A symbol, picture or word will do. Just above where the patient normally sits (if you consult in one space) or carried around (if you consult in different spaces).

And when you look at your space, even in the middle of the most stressful moments, you can make sure it enables you to feel belonging, safety, containment, awareness and empowerment too.

Sculpture

Beauty paints your form and highlights the space
Touch feels your warmth yet strangles the place
Where hope moulds our hearts and twists our soul
Love carving its shape and leaving its hole.

– JA

Chapter 9

'Effectiveness'

Activity 9.1: Evidence-based practice (30 minutes)

Think of a recent patient.

What did you do for him or her? Perhaps you dressed a wound, or prescribed some medicine, or carried out some surgery or manipulation? Write down what he or she was like before you did anything, then what you actually did, and what he or she was like afterwards.

Did what you did 'work'? Was it 'effective'?

Can you prove that?

Seriously, can you? Go ahead and actually try. Not in your mind, but with proper, written-down proof that someone else could look at and say: 'Wow, that really worked!' or 'Sorry, that failed.'

Not easy, is it?

As professional practitioners, we don't just practise. We also have a duty to monitor and evaluate our practice, to make sure it stays safe and effective. These monitoring and evaluating skills are important tools that we hope to master. But they can be tyrants too, if we come so obsessed by our outcomes that we forget to act in the best interests of our patients.

What do we mean by 'effective'? It's actually not so easy to pin down, but let's have a go.

Fortunately, the Hippocratic Oath has set the bar at an achievable level.

First, do no harm.'[75]

Unfortunately, the evidence is that despite this, not only do we sometimes practise ineffectively, we do sometimes harm and mislead our patients, and we sometimes waste valuable resources too, albeit unwittingly.

Some say that ignorance is no excuse for transgression, but that seems a little hard, as we cannot avoid ignorance. Nevertheless, if we are to be integrated practitioners, we hope that we can become aware of and then use practices that are as effective and harmless as possible. That means we hope to be able to test and demonstrate the effectiveness of what we do, to ourselves, to our patients and to our colleagues.

In that case, we might be rather disturbed to find that the news is not good. Some studies suggest less than 50% of 'conventional' practice and less that 40% of 'complementary and alternative medicine' (CAM) practice is either effective or likely to be effective.[76] What is worse, ineffective treatments and remedies are, counter-intuitively, more likely to take hold and spread in societal consciousness.[77]

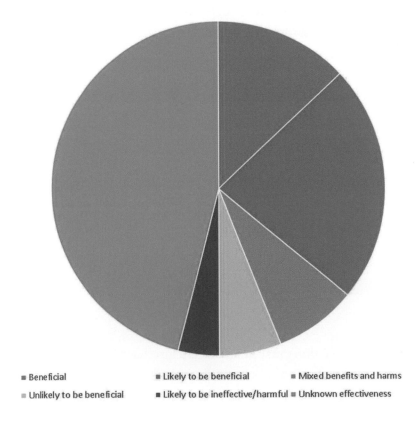

- Beneficial
- Unlikely to be beneficial
- Likely to be beneficial
- Likely to be ineffective/harmful
- Mixed benefits and harms
- Unknown effectiveness

This pie chart displays analysis by the *Clinical Evidence* subsidiary of the *British Medical Journal,* and looks at effectiveness (or otherwise) of medical treatments currently in use. It is a salutary sight.[78]

HOW DO WE ASSESS EFFECTIVENESS?

To be fair, it is not easy to prove the effectiveness of something we cannot easily define. As we have seen, both 'knowledge' and 'health' are very slippery concepts, so it is not surprising that 'effectiveness' is a very slippery concept as well. We have great difficulty trying to make endpoint judgements about what is effective or not.

Activity 9.2: 'How do I feel'? (30 minutes)

Consider the statement 'I feel great' (or, if you in a more downbeat mood, try 'I feel awful').

Can you prove that?

No, seriously, can you? Go ahead and try. Maybe come up with some evidence that an outsider could observe that would prove to them that you feel great (or awful). Or maybe come up with some evidence of the existence of feelings that you are experiencing that prove to yourself that you actually do feel great (or awful).

Now look at your proofs. Are they reliable and valid? Is it possible either you or an outside observer could be mistaken about how you feel?

There are three major problems in trying to answer 'effectiveness' questions about health:

1　Health is both objectively and subjectively experienced, but, as we will explore more in workbook 5, objective methods and subjective methods of enquiry generate different answers to questions of 'truth'.[79]

2　We can make knowledge claims about either the objective or subjective experiences of health, but we have to use different methods of enquiry to check the validity of any such claims. We can't use objective methods (also called empirical or scientific methods) to test subjective claims, and we can't use subjective methods (also called hermeneutic or interpretive methods) to test objective claims. So the method we use to measure effectiveness of our practice will dictate how effective we find the practice to be.[80]

3　There are considerable philosophical and scientific doubts that true 'objectivity' is possible or that 'objectivity' and 'subjectivity' are categorically different.[81]

In an integrated and relational universe perhaps all this is not surprising, but it is a startling idea for those of us brought up and trained within an empirical world-view.

> Often, when I point this out to students in the UK, they look at me with deep suspicion, as if I am saying something heretical. But in fact even the forerunners of evidence-based medicine pointed out the many limitations of their method, and the very great risk of an 'evidence-based' approach becoming tyrannical if poorly understood or used (*see* Sackett's quote below in this section).

Therefore, if we are to make claims about the effectiveness of any particular practice, we first have to own up to, and then justify, the particular perspective we are using (internal or external) and the particular method of enquiry we are planning to use (empirical or hermeneutical).

AN EMPIRICAL ENQUIRY OF EFFECTIVENESS

In theory we can investigate empirically any entities that consist of energy or matter. We can do that because we can sense them, either directly or by using technology. We are limited only by the ability of our senses or technology to sense the energy or matter of the entities in question.

By observing systematically, we can start to notice patterns and suggest hypotheses (such as 'all swans are white'). We then try to falsify these hypotheses by experimentation (for example, by looking for a black swan).

If we cannot falsify our hypotheses, we can become ever more confident of the validity of the hypotheses. In scientific terms, the probability of our hypothesis being false reduces. But we can never prove our hypotheses (because we cannot test every swan that ever existed or will exist for whiteness).

In the world of health practice, there are many entities that we can observe and test like this: the effects of treatment, the harms of interventions, the sensitivity and specificity of tests, the association between risk factors and illness, the nature and types of behaviours, and so on. For this reason, the empirical approach has been hugely beneficial in advancing our understanding of health and the application of health practice.[82]

Empirical methods of enquiry are very helpful in answering such questions as the following.

- Is treatment *a* likely to be more effective than treatment *b*?
- Is investigation *x* more likely to be dangerous than investigation *y*?
- Is lifestyle *m* more likely to be associated with illness than lifestyle *n*?
- Is behaviour 1 more likely to lead to outcome *x* than behaviour 2?

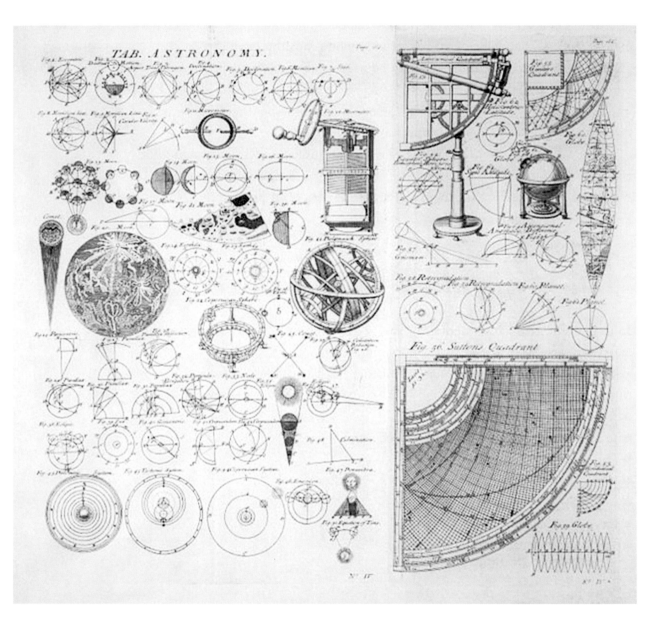

The stars – an empirical view[83]

AN INTERPRETIVE ENQUIRY OF EFFECTIVENESS

Not every entity in our universe consists of matter or energy, and so not every entity in our universe can be observed or measured.

Our experience of existence is full of abstract and conceptual entities, such as memories, thoughts, emotions and feelings. Our life is often driven by, and dedicated to, entirely conceptual entities, such as beauty, justice, truth, enlightenment and love. Feelings such as sadness, loss, euphoria, boredom and anger colour our experience, and go a long way to determining how 'healthy' we feel.

Indeed, 'health' and 'ill health' are themselves abstract conceptual entities. We cannot point at something and say: 'Look, there goes health!' Our sense of health and ill-health is a subjective one, and so one that cannot be directly experienced or measured by a purely empirical approach.[84]

Given all of this, it is not surprising that empirical and scientific methods of enquiry alone are insufficient for a full enquiry of integrated health practice. That's why we seek balance with an interpretive, experiential perspective, sometimes known as a 'hermeneutic' enquiry.

I feel as healthy as I am, and I am as healthy as I feel.

In the interpretive, hermeneutical world, we cannot say what something 'is', but we can always say what something is experienced 'as'.

For example, if I have a severe, persistent headache, I may interpret it 'as' many things, which might include:

- a result of scalp muscle tension
- a manifestation of too much beer the night before
- a punishment for past misdeeds
- the result of poor posture
- a visitation of malign spirits
- an embodiment of unresolved grief
- an early symptom of a brain tumour.

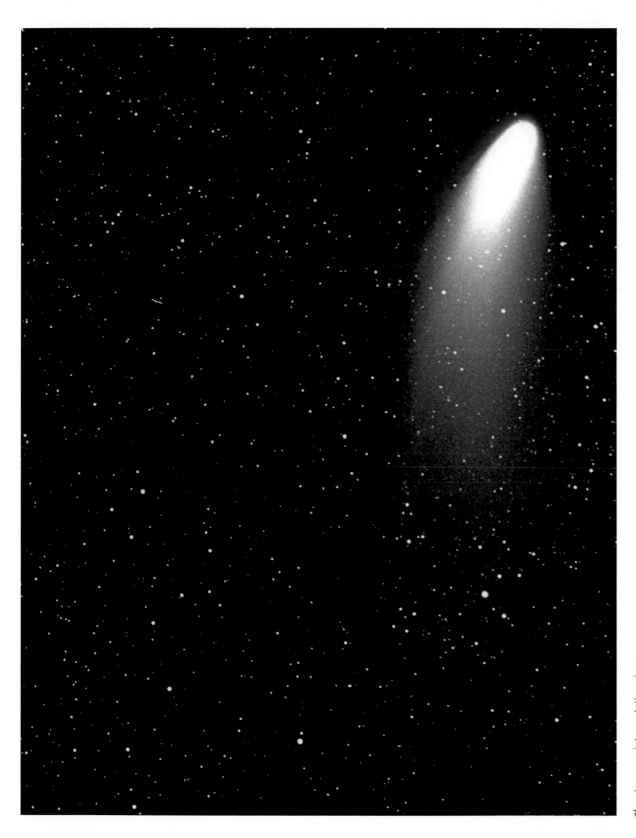

The stars – an interpretative view.

LOOKING FOR 'EVIDENCE' OF EFFECTIVENESS

If we are to find 'evidence' of our 'effectiveness', it seems that we need to look for both empirical and interpretive evidence of that effectiveness.

Sometimes we can measure effectiveness of our health practice by observing its effects on matter or energy. When we use empirical enquiry like this, we might wish to set about that empirical enquiry in a systematic, scientific way, to ensure any findings are as valid, falsifiable and generalisable as possible.[85]

Sometimes we cannot measure the effectiveness of our health practice by observing its effects on matter or energy, because the patient is experiencing health or ill-health in abstract or subjective ways, such as through thoughts, feelings, values, beliefs or emotions. In such situations, we can use interpretive or hermeneutical approaches, again in a systematic way.[86]

We sometimes get confused between the 'validity', 'generalisability' and 'falsifiability' of interpretive approaches. Interpretive approaches are valid. If I tell my story and give my interpretation, that is a valid interpretation for me. However, it is not necessarily generalisable to other people, nor is it falsifiable by an external observer. So interpretive approaches do not fulfil all of the criteria of the 'scientific method', but they are nevertheless valid forms of enquiry.

As integrated practitioners, to reduce the chance of harming our patients, and to improve the chances of benefiting them in some way, we are required to continuously question what we do. This is not easy, because both empirical and interpretive enquiries of effectiveness require systematic professionalism and effort.

It is less easy still when we come to realise that we can't simply fall back on one method of enquiry alone. We need to become masters of both equally, because health is both an objective demonstration and a subjective experience of existence. If we forget that, we will be less balanced and less effective practitioners.

> Good practitioners use both individual clinical expertise and the best available external evidence, and neither alone is enough. Without clinical expertise, practice risks becoming tyrannised by evidence, for even excellent external evidence may be inapplicable to or inappropriate for an individual patient. Without current best evidence, practice risks becoming rapidly out of date, to the detriment of patients.
>
> – Professor David Sackett, co-founder of the evidence-based medicine movement[87]

BEING WARY OF POWER CLAIMS DRESSED AS KNOWLEDGE CLAIMS

Knowledge claims are also power claims.

Health practice is very big business, and very expensive, so there are many different people and groups with interests in what and how we practise.

That means 'evidence' can be used by all sorts of power brokers acting in their own interests, rather than those of the patient. For example, the bio-pharmaceutical industry, the complementary and alternative health industry, governments, and (last but not least) our very own professional organisations.[88]

> And, whisper it quietly, but even we health practitioners have a vested interest in getting our patients to see things 'our way'.

As health practitioners, whose primary aim is 'first do no harm', it is right that we should take a sceptical approach to any knowledge claim, including (and perhaps particularly) our own. The onus is always on a new idea to prove itself over an old one; and the onus is always on us to be as skilful as we can be in using effective approaches.

Truth claims may seek to support their validity by appeals to evidence, or dispute other truth claims by seeking to refute their evidence. This is fine, but we can get sucked into fallacy if we try to apply the wrong method of enquiry to the particular truth claim. Empirical claims need to be tested by empirical enquiries, but they cannot be tested by interpretive enquiries – and vice versa.

What we can do is recognise that any truth claim should be judged against its own inherent mechanism for making that truth claim: empirical or interpretive. As practitioners it may be helpful to become skilful in both, because we are whole people caring for whole patients in a whole universe.

> So, if a pharmaceutical company tells us that drug X reduces mortality more than drug Y, we can say: 'Show us the evidence of benefits and harms, and it better be good evidence, because we will not risk harming our patients.'
>
> And if an elderly patient tells us he had a massage, and it was the first time for years that he had felt the comfort of human touch, and that it enabled him to cry for his long dead wife. We can think: 'That was effective for him.'

Activity 9.3: How effective is your practice? (1 hour)

Have a look again at the pie chart on page 88, and spend a few minutes reflecting on it.

Now look back at the last 10 or 20 patients you have seen, and list down what you did for them.

Next to each of them, come to a judgement about how well your treatment 'worked' and how you might go about 'proving' that effectiveness.

Now zoom back out. What tools did you need to use to prove the effectiveness: empirical or interpretive?

Go back to the list, and try to 'prove' the effectiveness of your treatment using the alternative tool, empirical instead of interpretive; or interpretative instead of empirical.

Finally, read through Professor Sackett's quote again. Consider quietly for a moment: are there any ways that your practice has become tyrannised by evidence, or any ways that evidence has become tyrannised by your practice?

INTEGRATING AND BALANCING APPROACHES TO HEALTH PRACTICE

As health practitioners we are relational beings stuck in a relational universe trying to practise a relational activity on other relational beings. We cannot escape this relationality by deliberately blinkering ourselves and deciding only one form of view, or measurement, or assessment, or judgement, is valid.

It can be quite disheartening to realise that, despite all of our training and experience, many of our beliefs, models and practices are poorly informed, of dubious foundation and of questionable effect. It can also be quite exhausting to realise there are so many other ways to practise healthcare, when we may feel only barely competent or confident in practising in the one way we have chosen.

But we cannot really avoid accepting that we have our own (partly culturally determined) values and models, and that these models and values will strongly determine which measurements, which assessments and which judgements we value most highly.[89]

What we can do is to try to become as aware as possible of our own ignorance, values and biases. We can practise mindful curiosity, keeping our eyes and hearts open, but always maintaining a vigilant and healthy scepticism (not cynicism).

Our job is firstly to ensure we do no harm to our patients, and secondly to try to do a bit of good for them too. The evidence suggests we do not always succeed in either, so a good starting point is a humble acceptance of that fact.

From that firm foundation we can begin to build our own narrative of health. What does health mean to us? What would 'better health' look like? How can we become more skilful in testing whether our efforts are successful or not? How aware are we (or can we be) about our own ignorance? How much do our own vested interests and egoistic drives distort our viewpoint and our practice?

Then we can start to ask our patients what good health and effective healthcare means to them. Why have they chosen us and our brand of practice? What would a good 'outcome' look like to them? How will they know when they have got there?

Only when we have done all this do we have any chance of practising 'effectively', because only then can we meet and address the concerns of our patients, using approaches that make sense to our patients, right here, right now, in our co-created present.

We can then practise not because we 'know' the 'right' way to practise. We practise because we 'know' whatever we do to improve someone's sense of well-being we are doing something that is compassionate, both for our patients and for ourselves.

When I Heard the Learn'd Astronomer

When I heard the learn'd astronomer,
When the proofs, the figures, were ranged in columns before
  me,
When I was shown the charts and diagrams, to add, divide,
  and measure them,
When I sitting heard the astronomer where he lectured with
  much applause in the lecture-room,
How soon unaccountable I became tired and sick,
Till rising and gliding out I wander'd off by myself,
In the mystical moist night-air, and from time to time,
Look'd up in perfect silence at the stars.

— Walt Whitman

Conclusion: integrated harmonic balance with the other

In this section we have seen how, whenever a health practitioner comes into relationship with anyone or anything, there is always a background of 'other' factors. These 'other factors' include an almost infinite number of people, things and ideas. We have looked at a few of the more important ones, such as learning, time, resources, space, knowledge, organisations, colleagues, regulations, targets, effectiveness, ethics, laws, appraisals, revalidations, and even space and the environment.

THE 'OTHER' AS TYRANTS

As we have seen in this section, across the world, these 'other' factors are a major source of frustration for health practitioners, sometimes leading to burnout, ill-health and occasionally even snuffing out careers. In this way, these 'other' factors may act as tyrants, reducing our efficiency, effectiveness and enjoyment in our practice.

There are days when health practice is like a soft pussy cat, happy, warm and easy to love. There are other days when health practice is like a tiger, on the point of gobbling us up. On these days, to survive, we just have to take a hold of the tiger's tail, and hang on for grim life.

Balance, therefore, is the key. But balance is not at all easy to achieve.

THE CRUCIAL IMPORTANCE (AND POWER) OF 'ME'

Therefore, before we go on to look at how we may be able to balance the 'other' factors that influence our practice, we might wish to remind ourselves that everything in our health practice begins and ends with us.

It is therefore of foundational importance that we put ourselves first, in a compassionate way.

Remember the universe in which we ex-ist (stand out) is far richer and deeper than the simple physical world of matter, energy and forces. Through our consciousnesses we exist in a universe of colour, texture, emotion, value and meaning. Everything we perceive through our consciousness is, quite literally, created by and experienced through that same consciousness. Therefore we create our relationships with ourselves and we co-create our relationships with other people. In just the same way, we co-create our relationships with the 'other'.

That means we have a choice: to create positive or negative me–other relationships. We have a choice to be tyrannised, or a choice to be in control, and use these relationships skilfully and effectively.

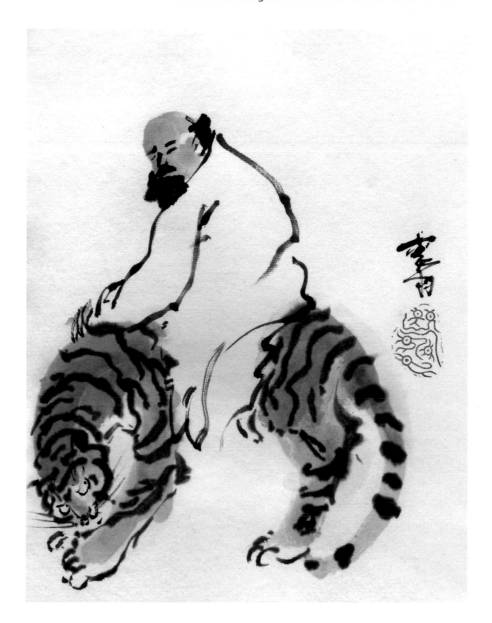

'Taoist Riding the Tiger' by Jan Zaremba, reproduced with kind permission of the artist. The signature is in the artist's name, Zaremba, transliterated into Chinese as Ch'a Ren-bo (a respected person concerned with that which unites human beings – compassion). The red seal, in the mystic taoist bird-script, means 'Long Life'.[90]

INTEGRATING THE 'OTHER' INTO OUR PRACTICE

If we choose to be in control of the 'other', rather than allowing ourselves to be in its control, we instantly convert the 'other' factors from tyrants into tools. This awareness allows us to achieve a healthy perspective. We have a great deal of control. While we cannot change those things which are determined by our physical nature, we can change our relationship with everything that we create within our consciousness.

This change sounds difficult and complicated, but actually it is a simple matter of choice.

We can choose which other factors to use and we can choose which other factors to ignore. The basis of this choice may be fear, or outside pressure, but these are not skilful reasons, and unlikely to lead to self-creations that are whole or balanced. However, if we choose according to compassionate aims, and according to our personal values, we have a much better chance of creating presents (and so futures and pasts) that are happier, more integrated and harmonically balanced.

To bring our choices to fruition, in other words to bring these choices to creation, it is helpful if we can be fully focused. We can bake cakes absent-mindedly, but we will be more likely to bake a delicious cake if we concentrate on what we are doing. That means that commitment and dedication to the creation of our choices and values are crucial.

As important as our dedication and commitment to our success is our mindful awareness in the moment. Whatever we do, whatever we say, whatever we create, it is always in the present. Therefore, the present is where we need to be. To become mindfully aware of the present we can remind ourselves, every time we feel ourselves getting distracted, to run a quick scan internally and externally, to discover which 'other' relationships are currently influencing my 'we' relationship, either positively or negatively, in the present.

So no one is saying health practice is easy. But we can at least choose which end of the tiger we would prefer to be.

When we are in the present we can, at any moment, look up at the infinite array of possibilities to choose those tools that we think will help us in our current task. Our choices are a product of our communication, with ourselves or with others, so it is wise to try to be as self-aware as possible, so we don't allow subconscious negative influences colour our choices.

When we have made our choices, it is simply a matter of drawing on those tools to start our self-creation, or our co-creation with our patients, remembering that the 'other' factors are our tools, not our tyrants. Like a painter choosing from his palette, or a sculptor choosing her materials, we can choose what we need to make the best self-creation possible out of the infinite universe of possibility, and maybe even enjoy the sheer, crazy pleasure of juggling many, all at once, and 'gathering paradise' as we do.

I dwell in Possibility –
I dwell in Possibility –
A fairer House than Prose –
More numerous of Windows –
Superior – for Doors –

Of Chambers as the Cedars –
Impregnable of Eye –
And for an Everlasting Roof
The Gambrels of the Sky –

Of Visitors – the fairest –
For Occupation – This –
The spreading wide of narrow Hands
To gather Paradise –

– Emily Dickinson

Activity: Bake a cake (time depends on your experience)

Mentally bake a cake. Consider all the factors that are needed. Try to be really pedantic. Think of every single one. The correct environment, ingredients, preparation, co-workers, utensils, stages, correct ambient temperatures, micro-organisms, chemical reactions, mixing, blending and sculpting processes. Consider the possibilities for error, for disruption, for interruption, for accident, for mess, for outcome, for likely effectiveness, for evidence of success, for resources and for workload. Allow the negativity to wash over you, to tyrannise you.

Now actually bake a cake. Get all the stuff out, blow caution to the wind, roll up your sleeves, and get stuck in. Enjoy and revel in every second of it, of the complexity, of the sensations, of the rich and deep smells and tastes, of the way the flour resolutely escapes, the miracle of how the sugar and butter blend into a cream. Marvel at how it raises, or laugh at how it doesn't. Sculpt it just how you want – in a fantasy of fluorescent icing, cream, jam, sweets and chocolates; or artfully and tastefully minimalistic.

Now sit down, make a cup of what you fancy, and eat it. You deserve it.

And if it tastes awful, go and buy one. The over-the-counter ones taste pretty good, and in my case, significantly better than my own creations.

Notes

1 The clue is in the title. Practitioners tend to be practical. While we might like to know the theory behind what we do, what tends to be more important is that it works. The original 'Integrated Practitioner' is a whole work comprising both theory and practice. This series of workbooks is intended to be more practical, so in workbooks 1–4 the practice will predominate. For those that are interested, the fifth workbook, *Food for Thought*, will discuss more of the theory that lies behind this work, as of course does the original book.

   However, for now, please bear with us, as there are 13 key theoretical points that underpin this work and without which it may not make complete sense. They are as follows.

   1. The universe, and every-'thing' within it, came into existence from no-'thing', and may presumably go back into nothing, and we can say nothing about the nothing, as there is nothing to say.

   2. The universe and everything within it (including ourselves) is entirely and intrinsically relational. Within this relational web, certain states of matter and energy 'exist' (stand out) with varying degrees of complexity (entropy) against that background of nothingness.

   3. Complex entities in the universe are holarchical. This means each level of complexity creates a whole which is greater than the sum of the parts. So, for example, clusters of atoms create molecules, clusters of molecules create cells, clusters of cells create organs, clusters of organs create beings, and clusters of beings create cultures and societies and biospheres. Each one of these can be said to exist on its own, as the interplay of smaller parts, and as part of the greater whole.

   4. Fascinatingly, and slightly disturbingly, we find that things that may appear to us to be fixed are also relational. These include knowledge, truth, beliefs, meanings and eventually health itself. Not only are they relational, they are also self-referential. For example, truth is a function of meaning, meaning is a function of language, and language is a function of truth. Self-referential systems always end up in paradox. It is therefore impossible to define with certainty what 'health' is.

   5. The universe is made up of the interplay between three things: forces, energy and matter. However, our experience of the universe is far, far richer than that. We feel warmth, beauty, taste, colour and texture. We experience anger, hope, fear, courage, joy and love. The reason that the universe appears so much richer to us is because of our consciousness. Consciousness takes in cold sense data derived from the forces, energy and matter of the universe, and uses them to

create the full richness of our existence. In other words, and in a very real way, our consciousness creates itself, and creates our experience of existence, as we go along.

6. While we think ourselves as having independent, concrete identity, this is actually just a matter of perspective. From a more macroscopic perspective, we are one infinitesimally small part of much larger relational systems: for example, our societies, our cultures, the biosphere, the noosphere, and the cosmos. From a microscopic perspective each one of our molecules and atoms comes from somewhere (or someone) else and goes somewhere (or to someone) else. From a quantum perspective we exist at the level of probability. From a cultural perspective the words, ideas and beliefs we use are mostly given to us by others.

7. When two conscious persons come into relationship with each other, each person's consciousness creates both itself and the other person. In other words, in relating to each other, in a very real way, we co-create each other.

8. Time does not flow. It is simply part of the space–time continuum. Our sense of time flowing derives from two things. First, our memory links together different states of existence in the space–time continuum in a linear way, giving us the idea that past flows into present. Second, our consciousness imagines future states of existence, giving us the idea that present flows into future.

9. This ability of consciousness to create past, present and future; to create itself; and to co-create others clearly has profound implications for what we think of as health, ill-health and health practice.

10. Health does not exist outside consciousness. It is a relational truth created by individuals, cultures and societies that has different meanings when viewed from different perspectives (for example, biomedical, psychological, sociological, or spiritual perspectives).

11. A common theme emerging from these different perspectives appears to be that health is something to do with the attainment and maintenance of a harmonic balance between different relational entities (for example, between molecules, between cells, between organs, between mind and body, between people, or between groups and societies).

12. While we cannot say what health is, we can suggest that health practice can therefore be seen as an attempt to co-create and maintain a harmonic, relational balance, not just for our patients but also for ourselves and our societies.

13. Being an integrated practitioner involves integrating all of the relationships and perspectives of our shared existence, using all of the tools that we have created and evolved through the history of human existence, to co-create 'healthier' states of existence from 'less healthy' states of existence. Health practice is therefore a science and a technology, but it is also fundamentally creative and therefore artistic.

That is enough of the theory. Let's get practical. After all, we are practitioners not theorists.

2 Edward Henry Potthast (1857–1927): 'Along the Mystic River'. Public domain art.

3 'Ars Poetica' by Archibald MacLeish, from *Collected Poems, 1917–1982*, Boston:

Houghton Mifflin; 1985. ISBN: 0395394171. Reprinted with kind permission of the Houghton Mifflin Company.

4 In the UK, the average length of a GP consultation is 10.7 minutes (Deveugele *et al*. 2002) which, rather coincidentally, is exactly the same as my own average consultation length. The NHS Institute has found that ward nurses in acute settings spend an average of just 40% of their time on direct patient care. Recent research by *Nursing Times* also shows that nearly three in four ward nurses say that is not enough and 90% of those polled say that patient care suffers as a result. In the US, the patient care activities accounted for 19.3% (81 minutes) of nursing practice time, and only 7.2% (31 minutes) out of a 10-hour (600-min) day was considered to be used for patient assessment and reading of vital signs. (Hendrich *et al*. 2008)

5 'Weaving the Weave' by master weaver Edwin Sulca Lagos, available at Artist Touch Studio at www.artisttouchstudio.com/?id=wpg18, reproduced with kind permission of Bette Endresen and Donald Endresen.

6 Various studies have shown the negative effect of time pressure on global job satisfaction, sub-optimal care, reduced patient satisfaction, increased patient turnover, and inappropriate prescribing. The main stressors in family practice in the UK include increasing workloads, organisational changes, too much paperwork, time, demand from patients, adverse publicity by the media, long working hours, problem patients, unrealistically high expectation from others, worry about patient complaints/litigation, insufficient resources, and interruptions by emergency calls. (Job satisfaction among general practitioners: A systematic literature review. *Eur J Gen Pract*. 2006, Vol. 12, No. 4, Pages 174–80 (doi:10.1080/13814780600994376). Irene Van Ham, Anita A. H. Verhoeven, Klaas H. Groenier, Johan W. Groothoff and Jan De Haan)

In nursing, workload, leadership/management style, professional conflict and emotional cost of caring have been the main sources of distress for nurses for many years. (McVicar 2003).

On the other hand, our job provides a variety of interests, we have choice in deciding how to do the job, we are involved in deciding changes that affect our work, and our working time can be flexible.

7 A system within which each item defines itself by reference to another item in the same system. So, for example: thought, language and meaning. Does thought generate language or does language generate thought? Is there such a thing as language without meaning, or meaning without language? Can truth have no meaning, or meaning have no truth? Does truth exist if it cannot be expressed through language or thought?

8 Gödel's theorem. We will discuss this more in workbook 5.

9 'seeker of truth' by e. e. cummings, from *Complete Poems, 1904–1962* by e. e. cummings. Publisher: W. W. Norton & Co.; Revised edition (14 September 1994), reprinted with kind permission of WW Norton & Co.

10 When we look inside our minds we find what is known as 'metaphysical knowledge', because it is beyond physical perception. Metaphysical knowledge is something that is directly and personally experienced through consciousness. We know that we are alive, and what it feels like to be alive, because we experience it at every moment.

Metaphysical knowledge is entirely unprovable, as it is entirely reflexive. It is also very difficult for others to 'know' what I 'know', except through the interpersonal communication, which is always limited at communicating meaning. Metaphysical knowledge is the foundation of the arts, and mystical and contemplative experience, as well as psychoanalytical (particularly Jungian) psychological practice. It is a fundamental form of knowledge, achieved through awareness and reflection on one's own existence. It is therefore the 'self' in communication with the 'self' (or indeed the universe in communication with the universe). It is not infallible, because it is very hard to separate 'pure' thought or 'revelation' from unconscious drives, memories or motivations.

11 When we look at things 'outside' our minds we can find empirical knowledge. This is knowledge of things we can sense and perceive. By observing recurring patterns in our experience, we can learn and adapt. From our observations we can suggest 'hypotheses' which we then try to prove or disprove using fair testing and logical reasoning. Some of these hypotheses become firm enough to be held as 'laws' or 'rules'. Empirical knowledge is the foundation of modern science, and the foundation of the 'modern age'. The scientific disciplines have given us incredible insights into our universe; as well as the technology to sense and perceive more deeply into our existence, to dramatically improve and also to destroy our existences. However, it is not infallible. We can only trust it as far as we can trust our senses, which can be influenced by our metaphysical and unconscious selves, thus giving us a 'false' picture of the 'reality' of the universe. At quantum level our senses may even influence what is happening just through the very act of sensing.

12 As relational beings in a relational universe we 'exist' at several levels (e.g. as cellular, organic, personal, familial and social 'beings'). Just as we can look 'inside' ourselves as individuals, we can look 'inside' ourselves as groups, such as families, cultures or societies. This is the world of 'constructed' knowledge, which tells us truths about what 'fits' in and feels 'right' to us? Different societies may use different ideas and language to describe the same thing (e.g. 'mental illness', 'madness', 'mental disability', 'possession'). Constructed knowledge is the foundation of social science and the humanities. However, without some grounding in 'objectivity', pure constructivism can become absolute relativism, which suggests that all truth is relative and therefore the value we ascribe to different truths is simply a subjective reflection of self-interest. It is also the foundation of the 'post-modern age'. It highlights the subjective and inter-subjective nature of knowledge, as well as making clear that knowledge and power are unavoidably intertwined (most knowledge claims are also power claims). However, without some grounding in 'objectivity', pure constructivism can become absolute relativism, which suggests that all truth is relative and therefore the value we ascribe to different truths is simply a subjective reflection of self-interest.

13 Deduction: Deduction is a process with which we move from first principles in logical steps towards conclusions and discoveries. We don't know where logic comes from, except to say that it seems a foundational feature of the universe. Deduction allows us to build very convincing and rigorous superstructures from first principles,

but we can never be sure of the 'truth' of these first principles because truth itself is mired in self-reference and paradox.

Induction is a process where, rather than starting from first principles and building towards a conclusion, we do it the other way round. We observe something, or some pattern, within our existence and we then work backwards in logical steps trying to arrive at first principles or scientific 'laws'.

Creation: Not all thinking is deductive or inductive. Sometimes we might 'see' things clearly, and ideas or answers may come from 'out of the blue', which we 'know' to be 'true', even though we can't really understand where they came from, or what relationship they might have to current 'reality'. How safe is it to trust these intuitions and visions?

14 What we 'know' is heavily influenced by the perspective we take, and by the tools we choose to use. Wilber (1997) suggests that different sorts of relationships and perspectives require that we ask different sorts of 'truth' questions (he calls them 'validity claims').

- From interior perspectives of 'me' we should ask, 'Am I telling you the truth or am I lying?'
- From interior perspectives of 'we' we should ask, 'How do my thoughts and beliefs fit within the thoughts and meanings of my family and culture?'
- From exterior perspectives of individual third person 'other' entities we should ask, 'Does the proposition correspond with or fit the facts as we see them?'
- From the exterior perspective of the collective third person we should ask, 'Do all the objective propositions make a functional fit in the overall system?'

Wilber captures this really helpfully with his table of relationships and perspectives.

	Interior	Exterior
Individual	Standard: Truthfulness (1st person) (sincerity, integrity, trustworthiness)	Standard: Truth (3rd person) (correspondence, representation, propositional)
Collective	Standard: Justness (2nd person) (cultural fit, rightness, mutual understanding)	Standard: Functional fit (3rd person) (systems theory web, structural-functionalism, social systems mesh)

15 David Hume (Hume 1739) was the first philosopher to point out that knowledge statements can be of two different types: 'it is' and 'it ought to be'. 'It ought to be' statements are 'prescriptive' or 'normative' statements made about what we 'ought' to do. Hume noted that people often try to say what 'ought' to be, based upon assertions of what 'is'. However, there is no logical link between the two.

He also differentiated between 'it is' statements based upon deductive knowledge (which can be safely arrived at through deduction), and inductive knowledge (which observes and makes judgements based upon observation). He made that point that inductive knowledge is based upon the belief that nature always behaves in the same way (so, for example, because water flows downhill today, we believe that it has always flowed downhill in the past and always will in the future). Of course we can never be certain that is and will be the case. So inductive and deductive statements are of wholly different types.

Hume's work had a large influence on the subject split of knowledge endeavours into mathematics (it is), sciences (it appears to be) and ethics (it ought to be) during the Enlightenment era.

16 Foucault was one of the first writers to demonstrate the close association between knowledge and power, and to emphasise the fundamental subjectivity and inter-subjectivity of all knowledge. For health practitioners perhaps the most important of his works is the *History of Madness* (Foucault 2006). In this work he demonstrates that approaches to the care of 'madness' are inextricably bound up with control and power of whatever the current, conventional morality of the time and location happens to be.

17 The term 'explanatory models was introduced by Arthur Kleinman (Kleinman 1980).

18 A quick overview of some common explanatory models of 'health:
- Biomedical models: which emphasise an empirical, 'scientific' approach to health, based upon research, naturalistic and biological explanations, the use of technology and surgery, and the use of physical interventions to preserve and restore health and to prevent ill health. This explanatory model is common in industrialised Western societies.
- Humoral models: within which health is seen to be a function of balance between different entities. Different ages and cultures have used different terms for these entities (for example, 'humours', 'elements', 'doshas'). Ill-health occurs either when these entities get out of balance with each other or with important external factors, such as diet, climate, the planets, sleep, enjoyment and so on. Healing is seen as a process of restoring a natural equilibrium by eliminating or compensating unbalancing factors. This model was originally described in ancient Greece and is common in Latin America, South and East Asia (particularly in Ayurvedic medicine), and is still fundamental to many laypeople's understanding of health in Western countries.
- Spiritual models: within which ill health is seen to be derived from personal or karmic conflicts with internal and external supernatural entities, which may be religious, naturalistic or ancestral. Healing is aimed at healing conflicts and restoring peace between people and supernatural entities and may use ritual, sorcery, prayer and atonement tasks. This model is universal, and is still predominant in African countries, but many patients use spiritual imagery, for example, 'I don't understand why this has happened to me!' or 'I don't deserve this!', as if illness is a result of the action of external, malignant power.
- Psychological models: within which health is perceived to be integration of conscious mind, and ill health perceived to be due to the disintegration of the mind (as a result of subconscious drives, conflicts, neuroses and psychoses). Healing is aimed at discovering these subconscious conflicts or traumas and bringing them into integrated acceptance and balance. This model developed with Freud and Jung and is commonly practised around the world, often alongside other models.
- Naturopathic models: within which we are all considered to be part of nature,

the whole of which is vivified by a natural force. This natural force flows through us all; when we are dislocated from it we become ill. By restoring or unblocking this natural energy, we can enable ourselves to be healed by it. Examples would include acupuncture, homeopathy and cranial osteopathy, but also commonly within 'New Age' approaches to health.

- Sociological models: within which health and ill health are considered to be socially constructed. They suggest that the way we define and explain our sense of health, and the ways that we express ill-health, are an expression of and so only understandable within the context of our own cultures and societies. So, for example, different cultures may use different terms to describe the same experience. We may use the terms 'mental illness', 'madness', 'possession', or 'breakdown' to describe the same thing, depending on our cultural preference.

19 'Spiritual Song of the Aborigine' by Hyllus Maris, was published in *Inside Black Australia: An Anthology of Aboriginal Poetry*, edited by Kevin Gilbert. Publisher: Penguin Australia Books (1 January 1989), but Penguin say that the rights have reverted to the poet, who died in 1986. I have been unable to track down the estate of Hyllus Maris so am including the poem as in the public domain.

20 Just as different perspectives (exterior and interior, individual and collective) can generate different types of truths, so different perspectives can give us different types of theories of health, for example the following.

- The biomedical model 'works' by objective observation and manipulation of the anatomy, physiology, biochemistry and genetics of the body, so it is effective when looking at health from the 'exterior' of the individual (i.e. what we can sense using our senses or technology).
- The naturopathic model 'works' by considering the balances of various factors within a whole system, so it is effective when looking at health from the 'exterior' of the collective ecological or environmental 'whole'.
- Psychological and individual spiritual models 'work' by listening to and interpreting what an individual has to say about his/her own experiences, understandings and beliefs, so they are effective when looking at health from an interior, individual perspective.
- Sociological and collective spiritual models 'work' by observing, listening to and interpreting what cultures, societies or belief communities say about their group experiences, understandings and beliefs, so they are effective when looking at health from an interior collective perspective.

21 Cognitive dissonance is the term we use when we find that we are holding conflicting beliefs or ideas at the same time. Instinctively, we try to reduce dissonance, as it is not a comfortable feeling. We may do this by pretending it hasn't happened, or try to argue ourselves out of it, or react angrily against it. All three of these reactions are commonly experienced when we practise healthcare. In fact, I would even go so far as to say that, if we start to feel angry or frustrated with patients, it is very often a sign of cognitive dissonance. For example, the patient who seeks then rejects help creates a dissonance with our sense of ourselves as 'people that can heal'. Or patients who get angry with us create dissonance with our self-concept as 'people who are helpful'. Or, quite often, we feel dissonance when our patients come with beliefs

that do not match our own. Perhaps, if we can start to recognise that cognitive dissonance is what is happening, and recognise it before our emotions or subconscious take over, we can start to use dissonance as an extremely useful educational tool. That's because dissonance forces us to revisit cherished, but unhelpful, beliefs and ideas and bring them out into the light, where they can be adapted and improved. After all, without light, how can we become more enlightened?

22 'Fractured Landscape' by Derek Toon at www.moonfieldds.com/art/fractured-landscapes, reprinted with kind permission of the artist.

23 Source: *The Poems of Emily Dickinson: Variorum Edition*, Harvard University Press, 1998.

24 From the 'getbetterhealth' blog at http://getbetterhealth.com/medicine-information-overload/2009.08.08

25 From Price DS: The development and structure of the biomedical literature. In: Warren KS (1981.)

26 The Guidelines International Network' can be found at www.g-i-n.net

27 'Information' from *Against the Evidence: Selected Poems 1934–1994*. Copyright © 1993 by David Ignatow. Reprinted with the permission of Wesleyan University Press.

28 In the UK the NHS has set up an 'Expert Patient Programme', particularly focusing on enabling patients to take more control of their own long-term conditions. Evidence is still quite thin, but initial studies suggest expert patient programmes result in reductions in GP consultations (7%), outpatient visits (10%), accident and emergency attendance (16%) and physiotherapy use (9%). At the same time they indicate an increase in community pharmacy visits (18%), health information service use (34%) and 'better consultations' (33%) among EPP course attendees. (Taylor & Bury 2007)

29 Originally researched in the field of consumer marketing, too much choice appears to be a source of confusion or frustration rather than happiness. What's more, too much information can lead to poorer rather than better choices, even though 'choosers' may feel more confidence and satisfaction with these choices. This may be because we 'choosers' are unaware of all the influences the information has on our behaviour. Indeed, a large part of our 'choosing' appears to be subconscious and automated. It follows, therefore, that as 'consumers' of information, health practitioners and patients may not be able either to recognise or skilfully use the large amounts of information available. Information in itself may not be enough. (Barry Schwarz. *The Paradox of Choice: why more is less*. Publisher: HarperCollins; New edition edition (1 Feb 2005), ISBN-10: 0060005696, ISBN-13: 978-0060005696).

30 Abbasi 2007.

31 'The World' by Paula Scher. Acrylic on Canvas. 1998. Reprinted with kind permission of the artist. More of her work can be found at www.paulaschermaps.com and a book of her work *Maps* by Paula Scher, is available from Princeton Architectural Press, 2011, ISBN-10: 1616890339

32 http://images.fineartamerica.com/images-medium-large-5/steampunk-information-overload-mike-savad.jpg

This is the essence of Marxist analysis, which itself was derived from Hegel's work on the distinction between oppressors and oppressed in society, at many different levels and in many different ways. Marxist analysis is not the same as Marxism, and it does not necessarily involve taking one or other political stance. It is more to do with the idea that humanity is in a continuous and dynamic state of interaction (or dialectic, or perhaps even conflict), with different individuals and groups constantly trying to gain or maintain power over others. Generally speaking, we health practitioners like to think of health as a relatively apolitical activity. And on the everyday practice level it may be so (although even at that level we may find some interesting perspectives if we start to ask ourselves whether we might be oppressors, or maybe even oppressed). At a higher level, health is an incredibly political arena. Around 10% of the entire world GDP is spent on health, so there is a lot of money to be made and power to be had. Therefore, as health practitioners, while we may try to be apolitical, we might wish to not be politically naïve, and try to be mindful of what is in the interests of our patients, and what is in the interests of 'others'.

33 Here's another one. This figure is what is known as a 'Cate's Plot' (after Dr Chris Cates, a family practitioner in the UK). I love these as they put into stark perspective the balance we have to strike between what's in the best interests of patients versus the best interests of other vested interests (in this case the UK Government Department of Health). The figure demonstrates the potential benefit of taking aspirin for a 55 year-old Caucasian British male (let's call him Jack), who is an obese smoker with high blood pressure and a family history of cardiovascular disease. It shows that if Jack takes aspirin he has a 24 in 1000 chance (in bookies' terms just about 50:1) of not dying because of taking the aspirin. The other possibilities include surviving even if he doesn't take aspirin (by far the most likely outcome) and dying even if he does take aspirin.

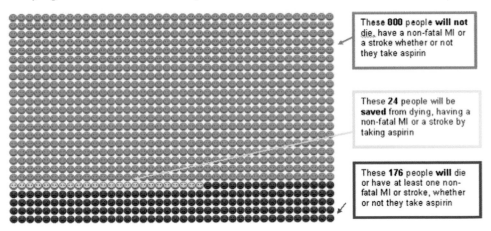

These **000** people **will not** die, have a non-fatal MI or a stroke whether or not they take aspirin

These **24** people will be **saved** from dying, having a non-fatal MI or a stroke by taking aspirin

These **176** people **will** die or have at least one non-fatal MI or stroke, whether or not they take aspirin

That is the empirical evidence. And it is very good, sound, valid evidence.

But with guidelines comes a sleight of logical hand. Guidelines take empirical evidence and convert it into moral assertion – that Jack 'ought' to take aspirin. However, as Hume demonstrated (*see* Chapter 2 'Health Knowledge'), this is not a sustainable logical link between empirical assertions and moral assertions.

These moral assertions may even be supported by inducements to the practitioner (in the UK, GPs are now financially induced to prescribe certain drugs in these kind of situations). This sets up a conflict of interest for us.

What Jack 'ought' to do is up to him. He 'ought' to decide for himself what he wants to do. And he can decide this by weighing up the evidence, with the help of his practitioner, and making up his own mind. If I were in Jack's position, I think I'd look at the odds, look at the potential harms of taking aspirin, and probably leave the drug well alone. But the key point is I am not in Jack's position. Only Jack is.

So where is the power claim and what is the vested interest behind the power claim? In this example, the power claim comes from a public-health, resource-constrained perspective of the UK Government. From its point of view, for every 1000 people in Jack's position who take aspirin, 24 people will not die or suffer a serious illness, and so will not need to be hospitalised. As aspirin is massively cheaper than hospital admission, even the fact that the other 976 people will take aspirin needlessly still makes economic sense.

It is so easy to get sucked in to the logical fallacy which is:

'Well Mr X, the evidence shows that A is more likely to happen if you carry on doing B [all logical and correct so far] and therefore I would recommend that you ought to do C [honk, honk, call the fallacy police].'

Whereas in fact the factual statement would be:

'Well Mr X, the evidence shows that A is more likely to happen if you carry on doing B. I can also say that, if you choose to do C, you have a 24/1000 chance of benefiting; and 976/1000 chance of not benefiting, and the government will save £XX.'

Then it's up to Mr X to decide what he 'ought' to do.

34 For every 10 questions posed, clinicians look for answers to four and find answers to three. (Ely, Osheroff & Ebell 1997)

35 We take information and we paint with it, we sculpt with it, using it to create healthier presents for our patients and ourselves. As we become more expert, we may find different techniques to use and create with this information, for example as follows.

- Prioritising: by reflecting on our practice, and particularly by reflecting on times we have not met our patients' needs, we can discover our knowledge gaps, and prioritise which areas on which to focus our learning. This process is called 'reflective learning' and is highly effective for practitioners, as it focuses our energy and resources exactly where they are needed. The idea of reflective learning has of course been around since the dawn of humanity, but it was described formally by Donald Schön (Schön 2002). He explained that everything in society is in continuous processes of transformation. We cannot expect knowledge to become or remain stable. He went on then to point out that societies, companies and organisations are learning systems, based on feedback loops. He also described how we all carry 'mental maps' which determine how we plan, implement and review our actions. When something happens in practice that our maps have not predicted, we first try to find an alternative way round the problem using the maps we have (he called this 'single loop learning'). If this does not work, we review the maps themselves, and alter the maps to accommodate the new reality (he called this 'double loop learning'). For practitioners, this theory brought learning out of the lecture theatres and textbooks straight into the consultations themselves. Thus practitioners can learn as they go, by reflection-in-action, and reflection-on-action. There have been subsequent criticisms of his ideas, and in fact later in this book we will be suggesting some significant criticisms with his 'reflective model' (and other similar reflective cyclical models based upon his theory). However, reflective practice has become hugely significant in health practice learning and supervision; for example, with Gibbs cycle and the PUNS and DENS learning model.

- Sourcing: one of the great benefits of IT is that it enables 'just-in-time' learning. Just-in-time learning is when we use tools to find the right information exactly when we need it, on demand. This reduces the need for, and the importance of, memorisation and behavioural conditioning, although of course we need a baseline level of knowledge even to know what we need to know and where to find it. As long as we pull together a range of sources that is relevant to our practice, we can pull up knowledge as needed and use that in partnership with our patients to co-create a new understanding and a new way forward.

- Evaluating: to be skilful with knowledge means being skilful with power claims. When someone claims to have some knowledge that would be useful for us, and particularly when they make the (always fallacious) claim that the knowledge that they have supplied means that we 'ought' to do something, we might wish to ask ourselves: what is his or her power claim, and is it compatible with my practice? What is his or her vested interest, and is it compatible with my practice? Is the knowledge claim valid? Is the knowledge likely to be useful to me and my patient in practice?

36 Self-care in chronic disease is seen as a significant element in managing resource demand and is also regarded as an empowering right for patients. Within the US researchers have looked at the most effective ways to enable people to manage their conditions effectively, using self-management programmes. These have been copied in other countries and appear to be very effective. However, the evidence is not uniformly positive, with some critics suggesting that it ignores the high dropout rates, that people who drop out are more likely to be higher need than those that stay in, and that it is just another way of extending medical power (and medical consumption) even further into patients' lives (Wilson, Kendall & Brooks 2007).

37 Photo reproduced with kind permission of Cytograft Tissue Engineering at www.cytograft.com

38 It may be worth spending a few moments considering why we feel so tyrannised by time and resource constraints. Perhaps it is partly to do with the way we see ourselves and our roles. Rationing sets up within us two different conflicts: role-conflict and resource conflict.

Resource conflict may come in many forms. For example:

- Knowledge: 'I could do more for this patient if only I knew more.'
- Money: 'This patient could really do with a week in rehabilitation, but the funding has been withdrawn.'
- Justice: 'This patient is getting a week in rehabilitation, but only because he can afford to pay himself, whereas the other patient, who needs it more, is missing out.'
- Time: 'If I just had some more time I could do so much more for this patient.'

Role conflict occurs because on the one hand we are carers, trying to provide for our patients' needs. On the other, we have to be gatekeepers, deciding what our patients can and cannot have. This role conflict can have negative consequences not just for the patient (who may be denied appropriate care) but also for us as practitioners. The conflict is stressful and it also puts us into competition with other practitioners, in particular with those from different disciplines or different health practices.

These conflicts generate dissonance, which we can find unpleasant, as we saw earlier. So we can be tempted to avoid them, or react angrily, lashing out at or rejecting patients or situations that trigger it. But dissonance is also a gift, because it is a sign that learning needs to happen.

39 Perhaps unsurprisingly, health practitioners across disciplines and across the world rank time pressure and workload pressure (which itself is a function of time) as the main causes of stress and job dissatisfaction. Also unsurprisingly, patients across the world also feel that practitioners do not spend enough time with them. We can slow time down, but only by travelling incredibly fast (many thousands of kilometres per hour) so, even if that were possible, we would end up very far from our patients very quickly, thereby defeating the object! Therefore, we cannot do much about the actual manifestation of time.

40 Gillon 1994.

41 Have a look at *The State We're In* (Hutton 1995) for an interesting discussion on how markets can work very effectively, but can also be distorted by vested interest and clever marketing.

42 Stephen Covey 1994 *The 7 Habits Of Highly Effective People.* Free Press; Revised edition (November 9, 2004). ISBN-10: 0743269519. ISBN-13: 978-0743269513.

43 MacKenzie (1972) suggests that 80% of our results come from 20% of our effort; whereas the remaining 80% of our effort results in only 20% of our effect. If we apply this 80/20 rule to our priority list, we can simply cut off the bottom 80% and concentrate on the rest. This may sound rather shocking, but, on reflection, it is clear that there is not much point spending time on unimportant, non-urgent tasks when there are always more important or urgent tasks to be done.

44 A good book to read about time management, in any field, is *The 10 Natural Laws of Successful Time and Life Management* (Smith 1994).

45 Minimising interruption is a variation of saying no. No matter how good at multitasking we are, being interrupted slows us down as we lose our single-pointed focus. This is not us trying to be saints; it is simply ineffective as it generates internal and external negativity that will continue to distract us now and then again later (when we have to make up to the person we have ignored or barked at).

However, it is not effective, efficient or compassionate to react by ignoring someone, barking at them, or otherwise being negative. To minimise interruptions we may find it helpful to brief colleagues ahead of time, remembering that, for that moment, the person requesting assistance becomes the owner of as much attention and empathy as we can spare.

'Look, this may sound strange, but I am really not good at multitasking and when I get distracted from what I am doing I get forgetful/annoyed/dangerous/panicky.

If you need something from me I will be sure to be available to catch up with you at XX.'

And when we get interruptions ahead of time, we can use exactly the same type of approach, say no, and go back to what we were doing.

And if we do lose it (as I frequently do) and tell someone verbally or non-verbally to p*** off, we can smile at our own weakness and folly, and make sure we apologise and explain later. It's no big deal.

46 Delegation is not the same as dropping responsibility. When we delegate we maintain a share of responsibility and we also take under our care the other person, to whom we have delegated. That means we have to act compassionately, honestly and effectively with them.

When thinking about delegating we might wish to check the following.

- Is the person capable of and ready to take this on?
- What support and supervision will I need to give, and can I give it?
- Do they clearly and fully understand what their new task is?
- Are they given the opportunity to say no?
- Which are the right tasks to delegate? (They should be things you can describe easily to someone else so they do exactly what is required.)
- Am I being patient, giving thanks and constructive feedback where necessary?
- Have I let go, and given them space to do it in the way they feel is best?
- Am I ready to pick them up if they fall, and encourage them to try again?

One of the great things about working in teams is that, even if there is stuff on my list that is not important or not urgent, the chances are there is someone for whom it should be important or urgent. If there is no one to whom this applies, either the team has got its priorities wrong, or the task should be junked (as it is ineffective).

47 'This is just to say' by William Carlos Williams, from *The Collected Poems of William Carlos Williams: 1909–1939*, Publisher: New Directions Publishing; Reprint edition (28 February 1992). Reprinted with permission of New Directions Publishing.

48 In 2009 only 270 doctors were called to committee investigations, of which only 68 were 'struck off'. Of a total population of UK doctors of 239 000, that is only 0.02%. While the commonest complaint is related to clinical practice, the most common reasons for being struck off are improper relationships with patients, indecency and dishonesty. Only 14 doctors were struck off for poor clinical practice or poor prescribing, which is a total of 0.005%. In other words, while we might worry about regulations and licensing issues, as long as we are honest and decent, we have very little to fear as our competency is well ahead of the bare minimum required. The UK General Medical Council publishes statistics (GMC 2009) of disciplinary action taken in the UK against doctors.

In the US study there was also a clear connection between dishonesty and disciplinary action. Of the nurses disciplined, 35% had a history of criminal conviction, while only 3% of the non-disciplined nurses reported such a history. There was also a significant association between having a history of criminal conviction and the rate of recidivism: the recidivism rate among those with such a history (56%) was nearly double that of those who had no such history (33%). (Zhong *et al*. 2009).

49 As an example, in the UK over the last 10 years, the government has focused on

reducing deaths and illness from chronic diseases. The main way it has done this is by financially incentivising practitioners to record and act on things like smoking cessation, blood pressure control, raised cholesterol, diabetes control and the use of preventative medication such as aspirin. These are issues that patients tend not to raise, because they don't (in themselves) make us feel 'unwell'. So patients that do raise them tend to be those who are better informed and educated, even though this group tends to be at lower risk. It is very hard to make sense of the statistics and variables, but it appears that there have been some benefits of this national project. Heart disease deaths, diabetes and hypertension control appear to have improved more than would have been expected without the incentivisation, but in other non-incentivised disease areas progress has been worse than expected according to trend. (DOH. *Delivering Care, Improving Outcomes for Patients*. Quality and Outcomes Framework, 8 February 2010)

50 For example, in the UK again, the success of the initial plan to reduce deaths from heart disease has led to the development of a plethora of targets, which are far more questionable in their effectiveness. The effect may have been that we may have lost our focus on the specific experience and problems of the individual patient in front of us; wasted time on targets that do not improve the health of the individual; or discriminated against patients with conditions other than those targeted.

One example is that practitioners should only diagnose depression by using a questionnaire called the PHQ; and that we should also always use the same questionnaire to follow patients up, but only between 8 and 12 weeks after diagnosis. Furthermore, to refer on for counselling, we also have to get the patient to complete anxiety questionnaires, phobia questionnaires, and social functioning questionnaires. The motivation for this, although dressed up as 'evidence based' appears to be largely financial, with the costs of care for depression rising rapidly. This rise, ironically, was largely caused by a previous campaign, by the Royal College of General Practitioners, to improve pick-up rates of undiagnosed depression in the community.

51 Mean achievement rate of 148 general practices for quality of care indicators from 2000–1 to 2006. (Doran 2011)

52 Initially it looks good: everything is improving, and performance in incentivised target areas improves significantly more than predicted by background change. However, on more careful examination it is less clear. Health outcomes seem to improve as a background trend whether we intervene or not. From that perspective, we can see that performance in non-incentivised areas improves less than would be expected by the background trend. So it may be that targets improve some areas at the expense of others, making little overall difference. This is an illustration of how targets can be both helpful and harmful at the same time.

53 Poem in the public domain.

54 In Handy's first book, *Understanding Organisations* (1976; *see* e.g. Handy 1995) he described how different organisations can have different cultures. In particular he highlighted the following.

- Power cultures: often based around a single or small group of very charismatic people who control the organisation. These organisations tend to function well in environments that are rapidly changing or in start-ups. However, as organisations become larger, it becomes increasingly difficult for the power holders to manage, and so the organisations either develop into another type, or fail. Small, single-handed practices are classical examples in health

- Role cultures: where members have clearly defined, usually hierarchical roles. These are often large, structured companies and organisations that are operating in relatively stable environments. Examples in health would be large hospitals.
- Task cultures: in which teams form and dissolve around particular challenges or tasks that arise. In the health setting these organisations might form, for example, in response to public health crises, or when larger organisations want to address specific issues (often using consultants to come in, address the issue, then leave).
- Person cultures: where there is only loose organisational connection between individuals who largely operate independently. Person cultures are quite common in health, for example medical partnerships, where each partner brings particular expertise or patients to the group.

In *Gods of Management* (Handy 1995), Handy uses a metaphor of the Greek gods to explain different organisational cultures:

- Zeus (power, patriarchy, 'the club' culture)
- Apollo (order, reason, bureaucracy, the 'rôle' culture)
- Athena (expertise, wisdom, meritocracy, 'task' culture)
- Dionysus (individualism, professionalism, non-corporate, existentialist culture).

55 Motivation is a complex and much studied area within organisational theory. However, some key theories are those of Maslow, Herzberg (Herzberg 1959) and Handy (see above). We have already discussed Maslow's hierarchy of needs in workbook 1. In brief, he suggests that all humans have a range of needs if they are to 'self-actualise' (that is, achieve and express their full potentiality). To be effective at work, we all need to find ways of meeting these various needs.

Herzberg's motivational theory is built on Maslow's theory, and suggests that people's needs can be actualised within organisations, but that people's needs can also be blocked by organisations. If an organisation meets our needs and helps us actualise ourselves, we feel motivated. If it blocks our needs, we feel demotivated. These are not opposite ends of the same spectrum, but on two separate spectra.

Demotivation occurs if we do not have enough of basic 'hygiene' requirements of a job: clarity of objectives, role clarity, working relationships, and reasonable minimum salary, safe and reasonably pleasant working conditions. Motivation occurs when we have enough 'motivating' factors: achievement, recognition, some challenge, interesting work, opportunity for growth, learning and development. Within an organisation that means we might wish to attend to each of these factors separately if we want to have a happy and motivated team.

Charles Handy's 'Motivation Calculus' (*Understanding Organisations* – Handy 1985) takes in the concept of 'meta-levels' that we described in the first section. That is to say, motivation is formed not just by needs and motivations, but by the interplay of these with the interpretations and assessments of those within the organisation.

56 www.opendoorcoaching.com.au/PDF%20files/Job%20Satisfaction%20Inventory. PDF

57 Organisations have six key functions. In a healthcare organisation these would include:
- design and delivery of healthcare
- finance
- human resources management
- communications and marketing to patients, contractors and other relevant communities
- administrative ('back office') functions
- learning, research and development.

58 Papadatou (in Amery 2009) describes the function of the health practice team as one which is built to contain grief and hold within itself the suffering of its members. When the team becomes unable to contain and hold the members, either because the degree of suffering is too great (e.g. when the team has been overstretched or dealing with particularly difficult or very many cases) or because there are problems with team cohesion (e.g. due to organisational or personal factors) the team can begin to split. Classically, these team splits can show themselves in a number of different ways.
- Scapegoating: where team members demonise an individual and project all their negative emotions onto him or her.
- Subgroup (or clique) formation: where the team splits into different subgroups, each with different agendas and values.
- Psychological 'splitting' of the team: a bit like scapegoating, but involving projection of negative emotions onto subgroups rather than individuals (i.e. where one subgroup demonises another subgroup).
- Change avoidance: where team members stick rigidly to the familiar, even where improvements are needed.
- Team burnout: which shows itself as poor morale, poor quality of care, chronic in-fighting and team divisions.

When teams begin to split, and conflicts develop, this has a serious negative impact on our sense of job-satisfaction and job stress of individual team members.

59 Organisations that provide health practice have a particular responsibility to provide support and supervision for their staff, and to ensure that the team is well managed. There are several organisational factors which, when managed poorly, can significantly increase job stress and reduce team and individual resilience. These are as follows.
- Work overload: every individual and every team has a limit to what they can do in the time allocated. Even the most efficient and effective team will get exhausted eventually. Good managers need to limit overtime and on-call work, ensure adequate meal breaks, and discourage 'stay-late' syndrome (which is common in health practice). Health practice work is not regular: there are peaks and troughs of activity. Managers need to plan not just for the average workload, but also for the extremes, and build in sufficient tolerance.
- Role clarity: when team members' individual roles are not clear, or not understood, or blurred, conflicts and burnout are more likely to arise. We need to know

the limits of our job if we are to set boundaries. Without clear boundaries, we cannot plan our time or energies properly.

- Loss of control: this is partly related to role clarity. When our work demands are outside our control, or where our managers are not good at listening to problems that arise in the team, we can feel out of control and fearful. Fear is a potent inhibitor of performance, and also a potent drain on energy and personal resources.

- Home–work boundaries: like role clarity, we need to know how long we are to be at work, when we can go off, and when we have to be on-call, so that we can plan our resources. We may slip into using 'family' metaphors for our team, but our work teams are not family groups (thank goodness!). They have different tasks, different roles and different rules. We should not blur the boundaries between the two.

- Resource constraints: these are inevitable in any healthcare setting. However, knowing that we could offer more to a patient if only we had more money, equipment or time is demoralising.

- Fear of job loss, discipline, bullying or other abuse at work: as mentioned above, fear is a very destructive element in health practice teams. Managers need to take care to create a supportive, non-abusive and encouraging environment. High-blame environments do not support good health practice.

- Change: high rates of staff turnover, frequent policy changes, and other changes are unsettling. We might wish to also remember that resistance to change is a feature of early burnout. The combination of the two means that managers have to take great care introducing and implanting change, ensuring that change is agreed with the team and that it is introduced within the abilities of the team to absorb it.

- Unrealistic goals: teams, like individuals, can set themselves unrealistic goals. Mangers also can expect too much. Good managers recognise the capacity of their team, build in some tolerance, and only allow their teams to fight battles they have a realistic chance of winning. Teams and individuals need some challenge, but not too much either.

60 If you have never seen it www.businessballs.com is a fantastic resource for anything to do with organisations and human resources.

61 There are a lot of good books about change management. One such would be John Kotter's *Leading Change* (Kotter 1996). Again, Businessballs.com has very helpful articles.

For information on clinical supervision in health practice, try Morrison (2005). There is also a very helpful series of articles online at the *Nursing Times* by C. Waskett (2009).

For information on how to run significant event/critical event analysis have a look at the article at www.patient.co.uk/doctor/Significant-Event-Audit-(SEA).htm

And for a good job satisfaction inventory go to 'Open Door Coaching' at www.opendoorcoaching.com/PDF%20files/Job%20Satisfaction%20Inventory.PDF

62 'Working Together' by David Whyte, from *The House of Belonging* by David Whyte,

published 1996 by Many Rivers Press. Printed with kind permission of Many Rivers Press and the Many Rivers Company.

63 From 'Creating a Therapeutic Environment', Diana Lalor, Psychologist, Counsellor and Psychotherapist. Perth, Western Australia. www.cottesloecounselling.com.au/diana_lalor.html

64 We all need some 'defensible space' or we tend to get stressed. At work, we may have little control over space, but if we do, it may be helpful to try to personalise some of the space, for example with a family photo, ornament or picture. Space is very important for our sense of who we are. This is known as 'place identity' and consists of our beliefs, attitudes, thoughts and emotions towards the environments in which we exist (Proshansky 1987). This might occur because we create memories of familiar and trusted environments and therefore start to develop attachments to them, just as we would towards familiar and trusted people. We may not be fully aware of this and may experience our place identity simply as a sensation of feeling comfortable or at ease, or uncomfortable and on edge in places that we don't feel familiar or safe.

65 At the turn of the 19th century, illness became coterminous with the body of the patient (rather than with the whole person). This meant that the body had to be taken to places where it could be more easily analysed, understood and treated. This scientific approach required a scientific environment rather than a domestic one.

66 Painted between 1658 and 1662 by Jan Steen (1625/26–1679). Location: Wellington Museum, Apsley House, London. Image in public domain.

67 Taken from 'Space and Time in British General Practice' by David Armstrong (1985) and available at http://kcl.academia.edu/DavidArmstrong/Papers/444201/Space_and_time_in_British_general_practice

68 Psychological research suggests that spaces that are 'therapeutic' are spaces in which both practitioners and patients feel like they belong (as homely and familiar as possible within the limits of the function of the space); that they are safe from harm; that they are contained (everyone's boundaries are respected); that they are informed about how to use the space; and that they are empowered to use the space in a way that is meaningful to them. Psychologists (Haigh 1999) have suggested that there are five key elements that go together to decide how therapeutic an environment 'feels' These are:

- attachment
- containment
- communication
- involvement
- agency.

'The sequence starts with attachment, the experience of which makes people feel they belong. This is followed by psychological containment so that they feel safe. It then encourages and expects open communication and demands involvement so that they can start to understand their place among others. Finally, it empowers them so that they feel a sense of their own personal agency and are thus responsible for their own feelings, thoughts and behaviour.' (Haigh 2002)

69 The way we 'fix' our space with walls and boundaries, the way we subdivide our

space with furnishings and plants, the way we use the individual space around our bodies: all of these vary from culture to culture. Fixed space includes things that are immobile (e.g. walls and boundaries). Semi-fixed space includes movable objects, like furniture. Informal space includes space around our bodies, which moves around as we do, and is determined by us. As cultures vary in all of these types of space, confusion and anxiety may get created between people of different cultures who use space differently to each other.

70 The amount of distance we like to have between us and other people is culturally determined. Hall (1966) described how different factors (cultural, sexual, social and individual) mean we all use informal (personal) space differently. Latin cultures use smaller relative distances and in Nordic cultures the opposite is true. Realising and recognising these cultural differences improves cross-cultural understanding. This is called 'proxemics'. Spaces can be either 'sociofugal' (space which encourages a sense of safety and belonging) or 'sociopetal' (space which encourages communication).

71 This section is largely taken from Lalor again, with some other inclusions from my own experience.

72 Professor Siegwart Lindenberg describes how we respond unconsciously and negatively towards clutter and mess. In a messy railway station, people sat on average further from a black person than a white one, whereas in the clean station there was no statistical difference. www.bbc.co.uk/iplayer/episode/b011mt0z/All_in_the_Mind_24_05_2011

73 In the UK, the Department of Health published a report into adult acute inpatient care which stated that that there is 'incontrovertible and compelling evidence' that patients find hospital care 'neither safe nor therapeutic', have 'inadequate arrangements for safety, privacy, dignity and comfort' and that there is 'lack of activity that is useful and meaningful to recovery (*Mental Health Policy Implementation Guide* – DOH 2002).

74 Time and space as concerns for social anthropologists derive from the work of Durkheim (Durkheim 2001). For Durkheim time and space have no meaning outside of the meaning mediated by societies and cultures. Therefore space and time are both personal and collective representations generated by, and therefore reflecting, the social structure of particular societies. Awareness of extension as space and duration as time is only possible by distinguishing different regions and moments and by encountering their associated boundaries and intervals. These divisions and distinctions have their origins in social and collective life.

75 The Hippocratic Oath (or at least part of it): 'I will use treatments for the benefit of the ill in accordance with my ability and my judgement, but from what is to their harm and injustice I will keep them.'

76 A Danish study showed that 68% of medical students use or have used alternative therapy, including herbal medicines and dietary supplements (50%), acupuncture (18%), reflexology (18%) (Damgaard-Mørch, Nielsen & Uldwall 2008). A translation can be found on www.vifab.dk/uk/statistics/medical+students+and+alternative+medicine?) (*see* Medical Students and Alternative Medicine, www.vifab.dk/uk)

In Uganda, where I spent two years working, it is estimated that 80% of the population never sees a doctor in their lives. This is not just to do with health beliefs, but also with cost and availability of doctors in rural areas. However, in my experience working there, even where conventional doctors were available and affordable, patients would often tend to take the advice of traditional healers over the advice of doctors (if the two sets of advice were in conflict with each other).

If we look at 'complementary and allied medicine' (CAMS), one study found that only 38% of treatments provided were either of positive effect or of possibly positive effect, while 4.8% showed no effect, 0.69% showed harmful effect, and 57% had insufficient evidence to say whether there was an effect or not. However, before we 'conventional' practitioners get too smug, in the same review the performance of 'conventional' treatments was not much better. Of these 41% were either positive or possibly positive, 20% showed no effect, 8% were actually harmful and 21% showed insufficient evidence. The journal *Clinical Evidence*, which is a publication of the British Medical Association, showed that only 13% of currently evaluated conventional treatments are likely to be effective, with 4% likely to be harmful, 8% a trade-off between benefits and harms, and 46% of unknown effectiveness.

77 This seems, at first sight, nonsensical. However, if we think about it, where a treatment clearly and unequivocally works, there is little debate about it and so most laypeople remain unaware of it (e.g. penicillin V has been the treatment of choice for serious streptococcal infections for decades). However, when no treatment works particularly well, fierce debate often rages, and there is plenty of room for new contenders (fair or foul) to find a way into the debate, and hence public consciousness. At that point, people start trying things out for themselves, and some may benefit, either through real or placebo effect. Converts, thinking they are on to something, trumpet their conversion, while those who get no benefit usually go quietly onto other remedies.

78 http://clinicalevidence.bmj.com/ceweb/index.jsp *Clinical Evidence* is a subsidiary of the *British Medical Journal*, specialising in using systematic reviews and evidence-based medicine (EBM) as a support tool to clinicians in practice.

79 We could decide assessments of health effectiveness should be based on measures of health outcomes. There are indeed measurable health outcomes, but, by definition, the only outcomes that are measurable are ones that we can measure.

We could decide assessments of health effectiveness should be based on how people feel. But we cannot measure feelings, for they are abstract entities within the conceptual domain. We can only ask people to describe their feelings, and then interpret them. If we ask people what makes them feel better, they may say a walk in the park, having a massage, watching football or having eight pints of beer.

In summary, we discussed earlier that we cannot use the same methods to investigate our interior worlds as we do for investigating our exterior worlds. The former can only be experienced, not observed, so they can be investigated only by expression and interpretation. The latter can only be observed, not experienced, so they can only be investigated by empirical, 'hypothetico-deductive' methods.

We can make knowledge claims about either of these worlds, but we have to use different methods to check the validity of any such claims.

80 In Chapter 4 we discussed the fact that, as conscious beings, we sense ourselves and the universe around us, but we also sense the fact we sense it (and sense the fact

we sense the fact, etc.). This means that we can be 'aware' on many different levels; from awareness of simple 'sense data' from our five senses, to 'meta'-awareness of complex and abstract entities like colour, love and beauty.

This multi-levelled awareness is sometimes simplified into 'exterior' awareness (what we can sense or our existence) and 'interior' awareness (the full totality of our experience of our existence).

This categorisation may be useful, because it reminds us that while 'you' might be able to see 'me' from the exterior, you can't have any idea of what it's like to be me unless I explain and interpret from my interior perspective.

But this categorisation may also be misleading in many ways, as in reality we can't and don't separate out our 'interior' and 'exterior' awareness and experience them separately. I can't simply see the electromagnetic radiation emanating from my computer screen I am now using without instantly interpreting it into an electronic 'page' with 'words' on it.

81 Quantum theory, Freudianism and post-modernism all suggest, from very different perspectives, that independent, objective, observers cannot exist. Quantum theory suggests that (at quantum level at least) the very act of observing affects the behaviour of the entity being observed (it collapses into either particle or wave form). Freud demonstrated how we have subconscious drives and motivations that undermine our ability to be truly neutral or objective in how we experience our existence. Post-modernism suggests that everything we experience (i.e. all 'reality') is constructed within our individual and group consciousness so reality is socially constructed, subject to change and subject to all sorts of power relations (both conscious and subconscious). However, for the sake of this chapter we might all feel able to accept that, within a limited space–time spectrum, and with certain tolerances for selection bias, subconscious drives and self-interested motivation, that it is possible to be reasonably objective and fairly independent of the subjects of some investigations in healthcare enquiry.

82 Although empiricism in health practice has been around since the Enlightenment era, it is really only in the last 20 years, with the 'evidence-based medicine' movement, that it has really gained the impetus and momentum that it currently enjoys. The evidence-based movement has brought great improvements to healthcare. We are more likely to use investigations and treatments that are effective and less likely to use ones that are dangerous. We are more and more recognising the value of prevention and whole population healthcare, rather that the 'see and treat' approach of my early days in practice. Finally, we are more likely to spend valuable resources to their best effect, rather than wasting them on ineffective services, investigations and treatments.

83 From *Cyclopaedia*, Volume 1, p 164.jpg. This image (or other media file) is in the public domain because its copyright has expired. This applies to Australia, the European Union and those countries with a copyright term of life of the author plus 70 years.

84 Take pain, for example. Relieving and preventing pain is a prime objective of all health practitioners. We all know what pain is, as we have all felt it. But none of us

knows what pain is, as it has no physical existence. We only know it by its shadows, its effects.

So to be able to 'treat' pain we have to know many different things about it, not just its nature, site, duration, triggers and so on. We need to know what it means to the patient, what feelings it generates, what fears lie behind it, how that particular person and culture expresses it and how pain is interpreted by the patient or his family.

85 In recognition of the finding that much of our practice is ineffective, a movement called 'evidence-based medicine' took hold in the 1990s, and has become firmly established ever since. Evidence-based health practice is only one way of assessing the effectiveness of our practice, but it is a very effective and skilful approach if used in the right context – for assessing the 'exterior' perspective of things. It is less possible to use it for assessing or valuing the 'interior' perspectives of health, and some aspects of health practice are not easily measurable or comparable.

86 One way we can do this is by becoming aware of 'themes' that emerge out of grounded listening to our patients; and then consider how these themes might improve our practice. Grounded theory was developed in the social sciences to look for evidence from hermeneutical sources.

In empirical practice, we start with a hypothesis and then try to design evidence to falsify that hypothesis. In grounded practice, we start with no hypothesis (although in practice it is doubtful that even the most professional researcher can approach 'evidence' without some agenda, whether conscious or subconscious). Instead, we just immerse ourselves in the hermeneutical data we have and then look for themes that emerge, gradually categorising and coding these themes, and eventually abstracting generalisable observations and even theories. These theories may then be amenable to an empirical approach, but not necessarily. The first application of grounded theory was in the sphere of health practice: in a book called *Awareness of Dying* which looked at data obtained from the expressed experiences of dying patients in the 1960s (Glaser 1965; reprinted 2005) which, incidentally, was the first study to identify how dying patients go through different stages of awareness of their prognosis, which is a theory that has held up and proved of great importance in palliative care.

87 Sackett *et al*. 1996.

88 A downside of the evidence-based medicine movement has been that, when combined with politics and finance, it has spawned a whole new phenomenon – health-related targets and guidelines. This is the appropriation of evidence by bodies with other power interests, such as budgetary, political, environmental or social interests. This problem was anticipated, although sadly not prevented, by Sackett and his colleagues. At the advent of the evidence-based medicine movement, a rather prophetic (if idealistic) Sackett stated in his article in the BMJ that: 'Some fear that evidence based medicine will be hijacked by purchasers and managers to cut the costs of healthcare. This would not only be a misuse of evidence based medicine but suggests a fundamental misunderstanding of its financial consequences. Doctors practising evidence based medicine will identify and apply

the most efficacious interventions to maximise the quality and quantity of life for individual patients; this may raise rather than lower the cost of their care.'

89 When faced with these tensions, we can make a few simple, and understandable, but nevertheless avoidable misjudgements.

- Putting too much value in one approach: the first is to put our heads in the sand, ignoring or rubbishing other models and approaches, and stubbornly carrying on with our chosen approach, irrespective of the evidence (scientific or hermeneutical).
- Assigning equal value to all approaches: the second is to assume that everything has equal value and that to question value and validity is somehow wrong. (That just seems inherently unlikely, although it is remarkably difficult to argue why it might be).
- Insufficient value: the third is to feel that one's own model, belief system and therapeutic approach is valueless, or less worthy than others.
- Multiple value: the forth is that we should all be able to do a bit of everything. We are limited beings, with limited powers. If we try to do everything, we will spread ourselves so thinly we will achieve nothing.

90 'Taoist Riding the Tiger' (11" × 14") by Jan Zaremba, from www.janzaremba.com. Reproduced with kind permission of the artist.

Bibliography

Abbasi K. Doctors: automatons, technicians, or knowledge brokers? *JRSM*. 2007; **100**(1): 1. Print.

Aked J, Marks N, Cordon C, Thompson S. Five ways to well-being. *Foresight Project on Mental Capital and Wellbeing*. New Economics Foundation; 2008. Web. Available at: www.neweconomics.org/publications/five-ways-well-being-evidence

Alladin A, Alibhai A. Cognitive hypnotherapy for depression: an empirical investigation. *IJCEH*. 2007; **55**(2): 147–66. Print.

Allen RP. *Scripts and Strategies in Hypnotherapy: the complete works*. Carmarthen: Crown House Publishing; 2004. Print.

Ambady N. Surgeons' tone of voice: a clue to malpractice history. *Surgery*. 2002; **132**(1): 5–9. Print.

Amery J. *Children's Palliative Care in Africa*. Oxford: Oxford University Press; 2009. Print.

Anielski M. *The Economics of Happiness: building genuine wealth*. Gabriola, BC: New Society; 2007. Print.

Armstrong D. Space and time in British general practice. *Soc Sci Med*. 1985; **20**(7): 659–66. Print.

Arnetz BB, Horte LG. Suicide patterns among physicians related to other academics as well as to the general populations: results from a national long-term prospective study and a retrospective study. *Acta Psychiatr Scand*. 1987; **75**(2): 139–43. Print.

Balint M. *The Doctor, His Patient, and the Illness*. New York: International Universities; 1957. Print.

Bandura A. Self-efficacy: toward a unifying theory of behavioral change. *Psychol Rev*. 1977; **84**(2): 191–215. Print.

Barsky AJ. Hidden reasons some patients visit doctors. *Ann Intern Med*. 1981; **94**: 492–8. Print.

Beating the Blues®. Web. Available at: www.beatingtheblues.co.uk (accessed 28 October 2011).

Beck DE, Cowan CC. *Spiral Dynamics*. Oxford: Blackwell; 2006. Print.

Beckman HB, Frankel RM. The effect of physician behavior on the collection of data. *Ann Intern Med*. 1984; **101**: 692–6. Print.

Beevers CG, Miller IW. Perfectionism, cognitive bias, and hopelessness as prospective predictors of suicidal ideation. *Suicide and Life-Threatening Behavior*. 2004; **34**(2): 126–37. Print.

Bench M. Open Door Coaching. Web. Available at: www.opendoorcoaching.com. (accessed 17 October 2011). Copyright © 2003 Marcia Bench and Career Coach Institute; reprinted with permission.

Berne E. *Games People Play: the psychology of human relationships*. New York: Grove; 1964. Print.

Betancourt JR, Ananeh-Firempong O. Not me! Doctors, decisions, and disparities in health care: how do we really make decisions? *Cardiovasc Rev Rep*. 2004; **25**(3): n.p. Print.

Better Health. Web. Available at: http://getbetterhealth.com (accessed 17 October 2011).

Black Dog Institute. *Depression*. Black Dog Institute. Web. Available at: www.black doginstitute.org.au (accessed 23 November 2011).

Blanck PD, Buck R, Rosenthal R. *Nonverbal Communication in the Clinical Context*. University Park: Pennsylvania State University Press; 1986. Print.

Blenkiron P. *Stories and Analogies in Cognitive Behavioural Therapy*. Oxford: Wiley Blackwell; 2010. Print.

Block N. How many concepts of consciousness? *Behavioral and Brain Sciences*. 1995; **18**(2):272–8. Print.

BMJ. How much do we know? Clinical Evidence. BMJ. Web. Available at: http://clinical evidence.bmj.com/ceweb/about/knowledge.jsp (accessed 17 October 2011)

Bohm D. *Wholeness and the Implicate Order*. London: Routledge & Kegan Paul; 1981. Print.

Bradford VTS. Trainers' Toolkit. Home. Web. Available at: www.bradfordvts.co.uk (accessed 12 November 2011).

Brantley J. *Calming Your Anxious Mind: how mindfulness and compassion can free you from anxiety, fear, and panic*. Oakland, CA: New Harbinger Publications; 2007. Print.

British Association for Behavioural & Cognitive Psychotherapies. Home Page. Web. Available at: www.babcp.com (accessed 28 October 2011).

British Medical Association. *Doctors' Health*. 8 May 2007. Web. Available at: www.bma. org.uk/doctors_health/doctorshealth.jsp?page=2 (accessed 28 October 2011).

British Medical Association. *Quality and Outcomes Framework, February 2010*. Web. Available at: www.bma.org.uk/employmentandcontracts/independent_contractors/ quality_outcomes_framework/qualityframework10.jsp (accessed 28 October 2011).

Brown D. Evidence-based hypnotherapy for asthma: a critical review. *IJCEH*. 2007; **55**(2): 220–49. Print.

Bruton HJ. Book review: nations and households in economic growth: essays in honor of Moses Abramovitz (Paul A. David, Melvin W. Reder). *Economic Development and Cultural Change*. 1979; **27**(4): 801. Print.

Bstan-'dzin-rgya-mtsho, Hopkins J. *Becoming Enlightened*. New York: Atria; 2009. Print.

Buber M. *I and Thou*. New York: Continuum; 2004. Print.

Buchbinder SB, Wilson M, Melick CF. Estimates of costs of primary care physician turnover. *Am J Managed Care*. 1999; **5**(11): 1431. Print.

Businessballs. *Job Satisfaction Inventory*. Businessballs Free Online Learning for Careers, Work, Management, Business Training and Education. Web. Available at: http:// businessballs.com (accessed 27 October 2011).

Businessballs. Web. Available at: http://businessballs.com (accessed 24 October 2011).

Byrne PS, Long BEL. *Doctors Talking to Patients*. London: HMSO; 1978. Print.

Campbell DT. Blind variation and selective retention in creative thought as in other knowledge processes. *Psychol Rev.* 1960; **67**: 380–400. Print.

Campling P, Haigh R. *Therapeutic Communities: past, present, and future.* London: Jessica Kingsley; 1999. Print.

Campo R. What the body told. *The World in Us: lesbian and gay poetry of the next wave.* New York: Griffin; 2001. N.p. Print.

Caplan F, Caplan T. *The Power of Play.* New York: Doubleday; 1973. Print.

Carroll L, Green RL. *Alice's Adventures in Wonderland; and, through the looking-glass and what Alice found there.* London: Oxford University Press; 1971. Print.

Casey PR, Tyrer P. Personality disorder and psychiatric illness in general practice. *Br J Psychiatry.* 1990; **156**(2): 261–5. Print.

Chomsky N. A minimalist program for linguistic theory. *The View from the Building: essays in honor of Sylvain Bromberger.* Cambridge: MIT; 1993. N.p. Print.

Cole SA, Bird J. *The Medical Interview: the three-function approach.* St. Louis: Mosby; 2000. Print.

Committee on the Use of Complementary and Alternative Medicine by the American Public. *Complementary and Alternative Medicine in the United States.* Washington, DC: National Academies; 2005. Print.

Covey, S. *The 7 Habits Of Highly Effective People.* Free Press; Revised edition 2004.

Cozens J. Doctors, their wellbeing and stress. *BMJ.* 2003; **326**: 670–1. Print.

Csikszentmihalyi M. *Finding Flow: the psychology of engagement with everyday life.* New York: Basic; 1997. Print.

Dalai Lama. *Becoming Enlightened.* London: Rider; 2010. Print.

Dalai Lama, Cutler HC. *The Art of Happiness: a handbook for living.* Audiobook CD. New York: Simon & Schuster Audio; 1998.

Dalai Lama, Hopkins J. *Becoming Enlightened.* New York: Atria; 2009. Print.

Damgaard-Mørch NL, Nielsen LJ, Uldwall SW. [Knowledge and perceptions of complementary and alternative medicine among medical students in Copenhagen]. [Article in Danish] Ugeskr Laeger. 2008; **170**(48): 3941–5. Available in translation at: www. vifab.dk/uk/statistics/medical+students+and+alternative+medicine?

Davison S. Principles of managing patients with personality disorder. *Adv Psychiatr Treat.* 2002; **8**: 1–9. Print.

Deber RB. What role do patients wish to play in treatment decision making? *Arch Intern Med.* 1996; **156**: 1414–20. Print.

de Girolamo G, Reich JH. *Epidemiology of Mental Disorders and Psychosocial Problems: personality disorders.* Geneva: World Health Organization; 1993. Print.

DeLongis A, Folkman S, Lazarus RS. The impact of daily stress on health and mood: psychological and social resources as mediators. *J Pers Soc Psychol.* 1988; **54**(3): 486–95. Print.

Dennett DC. *Consciousness Explained.* London: Penguin; 1993. Print.

Deveugele M, Derese A, van den Brink-Muinen A, *et al.* Consultation length in general practice: cross sectional study in six European countries. *BMJ.* 2002; **325**(7362): 472. Print.

Dewey J. *How We Think.* Boston: D.C. Heath & Co; 1910. Print.

Dickinson E, Franklin RW. *The Poems of Emily Dickinson*. Cambridge, MA: Belknap of Harvard University Press; 1998. Print.

Digman JM. Personality structure: emergence of the five-factor model. *Annu Rev Psychology*. 1990; **41**(1): 417–40. Print.

DiMatteo M, Robin CD, Sherbourne RD, *et al.* Physicians' characteristics influence patients' adherence to medical treatment: results from the Medical Outcomes Study. *Health Psychol*. 1993; **12**(2): 93–102. Print.

DOH. *Improving Access to Psychological Therapies (IAPT) Programme: computerised Cognitive Behavioural Therapy (cCBT) implementation guidance*. Department of Health, UK; March 2007. Web. Available at: www.dh.gov.uk/en/Publicationsand statistics/Publications/PublicationsPolicyAndGuidance/DH_073470

DOH. *Delivering Care, Improving Outcomes for Patients*. Quality and Outcomes Framework; 8 February 2010.

DOH. *Mental Health and Ill Health in Doctors*. London: Crown Publishing; 2008. Department of Health. Web. Available at: www.dh.gov.uk/en/Publicationsandstatistics/ Publications/PublicationsPolicyAndGuidance/DH_083066.

DOH. *Mental Health Policy Implementation Guide: adult acute inpatient care provision*. Department of Health (UK); 2002. Web. Available at: www.positive-options.com/ news/downloads/DoH_-_Adult_Acute_In-patient_Care_Provision_-_2002.pdf.

DOH. *The GP Patient Survey: general information*. The GP Patient Survey. UK Department of Health; 2010. Web. Available at: www.gp-patient.co.uk/info

Doran T. Effect of financial incentives on incentivised and non-incentivised clinical activities: longitudinal analysis of data from the UK Quality and Outcomes Framework. *BMJ*. 2011; **342**: 590–8. Print.

Dowson JH, Grounds A. *Personality Disorders: recognition and clinical management*. Cambridge: Cambridge University Press; 1995. Print.

Dunnette MD, Hough LM, Triandis HC. *Handbook of Industrial and Organizational Psychology*. Palo Alto, CA: Consulting Psychologists; 1990. Print.

Durkheim É, Cladis CS. *The Elementary Forms of Religious Life*. Oxford: Oxford University Press; 2001. Print.

Durojave OC. Health screening: is it always worth doing? *The Internet Journal of Epidemiology*. 2009; **7**(1): n.p. Print.

Easterlin RA. Does economic growth improve the human lot? Some empirical evidence. In: David PA, Reder MW, editors. *Nations and Households in Economic Growth: essays in honor of Moses Abramovitz*. New York: Academic Press; 1974. Print.

Edelman GM, Mountcastle VB. *The Mindful Brain: cortical organization and the group-selective theory of higher brain function*. Cambridge: MIT; 1978. Print.

Edelman GM, Tononi G. *A Universe of Consciousness: how matter becomes imagination*. New York, NY: Basic; 2000. Print.

Ely JW, Osheroff JA, Ebell M. Analysis of questions asked by family doctors regarding patient care. *BMJ*. 1997; **319**: 358–61. Print.

Epstein RM. Mindful practice. *JAMA*. 1999; **292**(9): 833. Print.

Eraut M. Non-formal learning and tacit knowledge in professional work. *Br J Educ Psychol*. 2000; **70**(1): 113–36. Print.

Erickson HC, Tomlin EM, Price Swain MA. *Modeling and Role Modeling: a theory and paradigm for nursing*. Englewood Cliffs, NJ: Prentice-Hall; 1983. Print.

Ericsson KA. *The Cambridge Handbook of Expertise and Expert Performance*. Cambridge: Cambridge University Press; 2006. Print.

Ernst E. Obstacles to research in complementary and alternative medicine. *Med J Aust*. 2003; **179**(6): 279–80. Print.

Evans R. Releasing time to care: Productive Ward, survey results. *Nurs Times*. 2007; **10**(Suppl. 16): S6–9.

Eve R. *PUNs and DENs: discovering learning needs in general practice*. Oxford: Radcliffe Medical Press; 2003. Print.

Everett DL. *Don't Sleep, There Are Snakes: life and language in the Amazonian jungle*. New York: Pantheon; 2008. Print.

FearFighter. Panic & Phobia Treatment. CCBT Limited Healthcare online. Web. Available at: www.fearfighter.com

Festinger L. *A Theory of Cognitive Dissonance*. California: Stanford University Press; 1957. Print.

Figusch Z, editor. *From One-to-one Psychodrama to Large Group Socio-psychodrama: more writings from the arena of Brazilian psychodrama*. Figusch; 2009. Print.

Finke RA, Ward TB, Smith SM. *Creative Cognition: theory, research, and applications*. Cambridge, MA: MIT; 1996. Print.

Firth-Cozens J. Doctors, their wellbeing, and their stress. *BMJ*. 2003; **326**: 670–1. Print.

Flett G. York researcher finds that perfectionism can lead to imperfect health. *York's Daily Bulletin*. Toronto, Canada: York University; June 2004. Print.

Flood GD. *An Introduction to Hinduism*. New York, NY: Cambridge University Press; 1996. Print.

Flynn JR. *What Is Intelligence: beyond the Flynn Effect*. Expanded paperback ed. Cambridge: Cambridge University Press; 2009. Web. http://en.wikipedia.org/wiki/International_Standard_Book_Number

Foresight Project. *Mental Capital and Wellbeing: making the most of ourselves in the 21st century*. The Foresight Project. The Government Office for Science: London; 2008. Web.

Foucault M. *History of Madness*. London: Routledge; 2006. Print.

Fowler KA, Lilienfield SO, Patrick CJ. Detecting psychopathy from thin slices of behaviour. *Psychol Assess*. 2009; **21**: 68–78. Print.

Frackowiak RSJ, Ashburner JT, Penny WD *et al*. *Human Brain Function*. 2nd ed. San Diego, California: Academic Press; 2004. Print.

Frankel RM. From sentence to sequence: understanding the medical encounter through microinteractional analysis. *Discourse Processes*. 1984; **7**(2): 135–70. Print.

Fredrickson BL. The role of positive emotions in positive psychology: the broaden-and-build theory of positive emotions. *Am Psychol*. 2001; **56**(3): 218–26. Print.

Gabora L. The origin and evolution of culture and creativity. *Journal of Memetics*. 1997; **1**(1): n.p. Print.

Gardner, H. *Frames of Mind: The Theory of Multiple Intelligences*. 3rd ed. Basic Books, 2011. Print.

Gettier EL. Is justified true belief knowledge. *Analysis*. 1963. **23**: 121–3. Print.

Gibbs G. *Learning by Doing: a guide to teaching and learning methods*. [London]: FEU; 1988. Print.

Gilbert DT. *Stumbling on Happiness*. New York: Vintage; 2007. Print.

Gilbert E. *Eat, Pray, Love: one woman's search for everything*. New York: Penguin; 2006. Print.

Giles J. *No Self to Be Found: the search for personal identity*. Lanham: University of America; 1997. Print.

Gillon R. Medical ethics: 'four principles plus attention to scope'. *BMJ*. 1994; **309**: 184. Print.

Glaser BG, Strauss AS. *Awareness of Dying*. Chicago: Aldine Pub.; [1965]. Reprint 2005. Print.

GMC. *Disciplinary Decisions*. Rep. General Medical Council. Web. Available at: www.gmc-uk.org/concerns/hearings_and_decisions/fitness_to_practise_decisions.asp

GMC. *Good Medical Practice*. Rep. General Medical Council UK, 2006. Web. Available at: www.gmc-uk.org/guidance/good_medical_practice.asp

GMC. *Printable Documents*. Summer 2009. Web. Available at: www.gmc-uk.org/concerns/printable_documents.asp

Goldberg LR. The structure of phenotypic personality traits. *Am Psychol*. 1993; **48**: 26–34. Print.

GP Online. *A Registrar Survival Guide . . . setting up your consulting room*. GP Online. 2010. Web. Available at: www.gponline.com/Education/article/1037805/a-registrar-survival-guide-setting-consulting-room (accessed 4 November 2010).

GP Training Net. *Consultation Theory*. Web. Available at: http://gptraining.net (accessed 12 November 2011).

Grant J, Crawley J. *Transference and Projection: mirrors to the self*. Buckingham: Open University; 2002. Print.

Greene B. *The Elegant Universe: superstrings, hidden dimensions, and the quest for the ultimate theory*. London: Vintage; 2005. Print.

Greenhalgh T, Hurwitz B, editors. *Narrative Based Medicine: dialogue and discourse in clinical practice*. London: BMJ; 2002. Print.

Grimshaw GM, Stanton T. Tobacco cessation interventions for young people. *Cochrane Database Syst Rev*. 2006; **4**: CD003289. Print.

Haigh R. Modern milieux: therapeutic community solutions to acute ward problems. *The Psychiatrist*. 2002; **26**: 380–2. Print.

Haigh R. The quintessence of a therapeutic environment: five universal qualities. In: Campling P, Haigh R, editors. *Therapeutic Communities: past, present and future*. London: Jessica Kingsley; 1999. pp. 246–57. Print.

Hakeda YS. *Kukai: major works*. New York: Columbia University Press; 1972. Print.

Hall ET. *The Hidden Dimension*. Garden City, NY: Doubleday; 1966. Print.

Hammond DC. Review of the efficacy of clinical hypnosis with headaches and migraines. *IJCEH*. 2007; **55**(2): 207–19. Print.

Handy CB. *Gods of Management: the changing work of organizations*. New York: Oxford University Press; 1995. Print.

Handy CB. *Understanding Organisations*. Harmondsworth, Middlesex: Penguin; [1976] 1985. Print.

Hawking SW. *A Brief History of Time: from the big bang to black holes*. Toronto: Bantam; 1988. Print.

Health Foundation. *Evidence: helping people help themselves. A review of the evidence considering whether it is worthwhile to support self-management*. Health Foundation; May 2011. Web. Available at: www.health.org.uk/publications/evidence-helping-people-help-themselves

Health Talk Online. *Shared Decision Making*. Healthtalkonline. DOH. Web. Available at: www.healthtalkonline.org/Improving_health_care/shared_decision_making (accessed April 2011).

Hecht MA, LaFrance M. How (fast) can I help you? Tone of voice and telephone operator efficiency in interactions. *J Appl Soc Psychol*. 1995; **25**(23): 2086–98. Print.

Hélie S, Sun R. Incubation, insight, and creative problem solving: a unified theory and a connectionist model. *Psychol Rev*. 2010; **117**(3): 994–1024. Print.

Helman CG. Disease versus illness in general practice. *J R Coll Gen Pract*. 1981; **31**: 548–62. Print.

Hendrich A, Chow MP, Skierczynski BA, Lu Z. A 36-hospital time and motion study: how do medical-surgical nurses spend their time? *Perm J*. 2008; **12**(3): 25–34. Print.

Henning K, Ey S, Shaw D. Perfectionism, the impostor phenomenon and psychological adjustment in medical, dental, nursing and pharmacy students. *Med Educ*. 1998; **32**(5): 456–64. Print.

Hermans HJM, Gieser T. *Handbook of Dialogical Self Theory*. Cambridge: Cambridge University Press; 2011. Print.

Hermans HJM, Kempen HJG. *The Dialogical Self: meaning as movement*. San Diego: Academic; 1993. Print.

Heron J. A six-category intervention analysis. *Br J Guidance & Counselling*. 1976; **4**(2): 143–55. Print.

Herzberg F. *The Motivation to Work*. New York: Wiley; 1959. Print.

Hinduism Today. *Join the Hindu Renaissance*. Hinduism Today Magazine. Web. Available at: www.hinduismtoday.com (accessed 14 November 2011).

Hilbert D, Cohn-Vossen S. *Geometry and the Imagination*. 2nd ed. London: Chelsea Publishing Company; 1990. Print.

Hofstadter DR. *Gödel, Escher, Bach*. Harmondsworth: Penguin; 1980. Print.

Hume D. *A Treatise of Human Nature; being an attempt to introduce the experimental method of reasoning into moral subjects*. Cleveland: World Pub.; [1739] 1962. Print.

Hutton W. *The State We're In*. London: Jonathan Cape; 1995. Print.

Hymes J. editor. *The Child under Six*. London: Consortium; 1994. Print.

Ignatow D. *Against the Evidence: selected poems, 1934–1994*. [Middletown, Conn.]: Wesleyan University Press; 1993. Print.

Internet Encyclopedia of Philosophy. *Time*. Internet Encyclopedia of Philosophy. Web. Available at: www.iep.utm.edu/time (accessed 14 November 2011).

Isaksen SG, Treffinger DJ. *Creative Problem Solving: the basic course*. Buffalo, NY: Bearly; 1985. Print.

Isen A, Daubman KA, Nowicki GP. Positive affect facilitates creative problem solving. *J Pers Soc Psychol*. 1987; **52**(6): 1122–31. Print.

Ivancevich JM, Matteson MT. Stress and work: a managerial perspective. In: Quick JC, Bhagat RS, Dalton JE, Quick JD, editors. *Work Stress: health care systems in the workplace*. New York: Praeger; 1980. pp. 27–49. Print.

James W. *The Principles of Psychology*. Charleston, SC: BiblioLife; 2010. Print.

Juran JM, Gryna FM. *Juran's Quality Control Handbook*. New York: McGraw-Hill; 1988. Print.

Kabat-Zinn J. *Full Catastrophe Living: using the wisdom of your body and mind to face stress, pain, and illness*. New York, NY: Dell Pub., a Division of Bantam Doubleday Dell Pub. Group; 1991. Print.

Kahn RL, Byosiere P. Stress in organizations. In: Dunnette MD, Hough LM, editors. *Handbook of Industrial and Organizational Psychology, Vol. 3*. Palo Alto, CA: Consulting Psychologists Press; 1992. pp. 571–650. Print.

Kahneman D. *Thinking, Fast and Slow*. New York: Penguin; 2012. Print.

Kandel ER, Schwartz JM, Jessell TM. *Principles of Neural Science*. New York: McGraw-Hill, Health Professions Division; 2000. Print.

Kant I. *Groundwork for the Metaphysics of Morals*. New Haven: Yale University Press; 2002. Print.

Kaufman JC, Beghetto RA. Beyond big and little: the Four C Model of Creativity. *Rev Gen Psychology*. 2009; **13**: 1–12. Print.

Keating T. Centering Prayer. Web. Available at: www.centeringprayer.com (accessed 12 November 2011).

King LS. *Medical Thinking: a historical preface*. Princeton, NJ: Princeton University Press; 1982. Print.

Kleinke CL, Peterson TR, Rutledge TR. Effects of self-generated facial expressions on mood. *J Pers Soc Psychol*. 1998; **74**(1): 272–9. Print.

Kleinman A. *Patients and Healers in the Context of Culture: an exploration of the borderland between anthropology, medicine, and psychiatry*. Berkeley: University of California; 1980. Print.

Ko U. Ananda. *Beyond Self: 108 Korean Zen poems*. Berkeley, CA: Parallax; 1997. Print.

Koch R. *The Natural Laws of Business: applying the theories of Darwin, Einstein, and Newton to achieve business success*. New York: Currency/Doubleday; 2001. Print.

Koestler A. *The Ghost in the Machine*. London: Hutchinson; 1967. Print.

Kolb DA. *Experiential Learning: experience as the source of learning and development*. Englewood Cliffs, NJ: Prentice-Hall; 1984. Print.

Kornfield J. *Buddha's Little Instruction Book*. London: Rider & Co; 1996. Print.

Kotter JP. *Leading Change*. Boston, MA: Harvard Business School; 1996. Print.

Kumar M. *Quantum: Einstein, Bohr, and the great debate about the nature of reality*. New York: W.W. Norton; 2009. Print.

Kurtz SM, Silverman J, Draper J. *Teaching and Learning Communication Skills in Medicine*. Oxford: Radcliffe Publishing; 2005. Print.

Lalor D. *Creating a Therapeutic Environment. Counselling in Perth, Western Australia*. Cottesloe Counselling Centre. Web. Available at: www.cottesloecounselling.com.au (accessed 24 October 2011).

Lazarus RS, Folkman S. *Stress, Appraisal, and Coping*. New York: Springer; 1984.

Bibliography

Launer J. *Narrative-based Primary Care: a practical guide*. Oxford: Radcliffe Medical Press; 2002. Print.

Légaré F, Ratté S, Stacey D, *et al*. Interventions for improving the adoption of shared decision making by healthcare professionals. *Cochrane Database Syst Rev.* 2011; **10**: CD001431. Web.

Lehrer J. *Imagine: how creativity works*. Edinburgh: Canongate; 2012. Print.

Levensky E, Forcehimes A, Beitz K. Motivational interviewing: an evidence-based approach to counseling helps patients follow treatment recommendations. *Am J Nurs.* 2007; **107**(10): 50–8. Print.

Lewin S, Skea Z, Entwistle V, *et al*. Effects of interventions to promote a patient-centred approach in clinical consultations. *Cochrane Database Syst Rev.* 2001; **4**: CD00326. Web.

Lewin SA, Skea Z, Entwistle VA, *et al*. Interventions for providers to promote a patient-centred approach in clinical consultations. *Cochrane Database Syst Rev.* 2012; **12**: CD003267. Print.

Linehan M. *Cognitive Behavioural Treatment of Borderline Personality Disorder*. London: Guildford; 1993. Print.

Linn LS, Yager J, Cope D, Leake B. Health status, job satisfaction, job stress, and life satisfaction among academic and clinical faculty. *JAMA.* 1985; **254**(19): 2775–82. Print.

Living Life to the Full. *Free Online Skills Course*. Living Life to the Full. Web. Available at: www.llttf.com (accessed 28 October 2011).

Locke J, Bassett T, Holt E. *An Essay Concerning Humane Understanding: in four books*. London: Printed by Eliz. Holt for Thomas Basset; 1690. Print.

Mackenzie RA. *The Time Trap*. New York: AMACOM; 1972. Print.

Maslach C, Schaufeli W, Leiter M. Job burnout. *Annu Rev Psychol.* 2001; **52**: 397–422. Web.

Maslow AH. A theory of human motivation. *Psychol Rev.* 1943; **50**(4): 370–96. Print.

Maslow AH. *The Farther Reaches of Human Nature*. New York: Penguin; 1976. Print.

May R. *The Courage to Create*. London: Collins; 1976. Print.

McCambridge J. Motivational interviewing is equivalent to more intensive treatment, superior to placebo, and will be tested more widely. *Evidence-Based Mental Health.* 2004. **7**(2): 52. Print.

McKinlay JB, Potter DA, Feldman DA. Non-medical influences on medical decision-making. *Soc Sci Med.* 1996; **42**(5): 769–76. Print.

McQuaid JR, Carmona PE. *Peaceful Mind: using mindfulness and cognitive behavioral psychology to overcome depression*. Oakland, CA: New Harbinger; 2004. Print.

McVicar A. Workplace stress in nursing: a literature review. *J Adv Nurs.* 2003; **44**(6): 633–42. Print.

Melville A. Job satisfaction in general practice: implications for prescribing. *Soc Sci Med. Part A: Medical Psychology & Medical Sociology.* 1980; **14**(6): 495–9. Print.

Mitchley SE. The medical interview: the three-function approach. *Postgrad Med J.* 1992; **68**(799): 397–8. Print.

MoodGYM. Welcome. Web. Available at: www.moodgym.anu.edu.au (accessed 28 October 2011).

Moran P. *Antisocial Personality Disorder*. London: Gaskell; 1999. Print.

Morrison T. *Staff Supervision in Social Care: making a real difference for staff and service users*. Brighton: Pavilion; 2005. Print.

National Institute for Health and Care Excellence. *Anxiety: management of anxiety (panic disorder, with or without agoraphobia, and generalised anxiety disorder) in adults in primary, secondary and community care*. NICE. March 2011. Web. Available at: http://guidance.nice.org.uk/CG22

National Institute for Health and Care Excellence. *Brief Interventions and Referral for Smoking Cessation in Primary Care and Other Settings*. NICE. 2006. Web. Available at: www.nice.org.uk/nicemedia/pdf/SMOKING-ALS2_FINAL.pdf

National Institute for Health and Care Excellence. *Cognitive Behavioural Therapy for the Management of Common Mental Health Problems*. NICE. December 2010. Web. Available at: www.nice.org.uk/usingguidance/commissioningguides/cognitivebehavioural therapyservice/cbt.jsp

National Institute for Health and Care Excellence. *Computerised Cognitive Behaviour Therapy for Depression and Anxiety: review of Technology Appraisal 51*. NICE. February 2006. Web. Available at: www.nice.org.uk/nicemedia/pdf/TA097guidance.pdf

Neighbour R. *The Inner Consultation: how to develop an effective and intuitive consulting style*. Lancaster: MTP; 1987. Print.

NHS Centre for Reviews. *Effectiveness Matters: counselling in primary care*. 2001; **5**(2): n.p. Print.

NHS Direct. *Decision Aids*. NHS Direct. Web. Available at: www.nhsdirect.nhs.uk/decisionaids.

NHS Institute for Innovation and Improvement. *Releasing Time to Care: the productive ward*. 2007. Available at: www.institute.nhs.uk/quality_and_value/productivity_series/productive_ward.html.

Noonuccal, Oodgeroo. *My People*. 3rd ed. Milton, QA: The Jacaranda Press; 1990. Print.

Ogedegbe G. Labeling and hypertension: it is time to intervene on its negative consequences. *Hypertension*. 2010; **56**(3): 344–5. Print.

O'Hara LA. Creativity and intelligence. In: Sternberg RJ, editor. *Handbook of Creativity*. Cambridge University Press; 1999. Print.

Open Door Coaching. *Job Satisfaction Inventory*. Open Door Coaching. Web. Available at: www.opendoorcoaching.com/PDF%20files/Job%20Satisfaction%20Inventory.PDF (accessed 24 October 2011).

Orwell G. *Nineteen Eighty-four, a novel*. New York: Harcourt, Brace; 1949. Print.

'Overcoming' series. Constable & Robinson Publishers. Web. Available at: www.overcoming.co.uk

Paice E, Moss F. How important are role models in making good doctors. *BMJ*. 2002; **325**: 707. Print.

Patient.co.uk. *Significant Event Analysis*. Health Information and Advice, Medicines Guide, Patient.co.uk. Web. Available at: http://patient.co.uk (accessed 24 October 2011).

Patrick CJ, Craig KD, Prkachin KM. Observer judgments of acute pain: facial action determinants. *J Pers Soc Psych*. 1986; **50**(6): 1291–8. Print.

Pendleton D, Schofield T, Tate P, Havelock P. *The Consultation: an approach to learning and teaching*. Oxford: Oxford University Press; 1984. Print.

Bibliography

Penrose R. *The Emperor's New Mind: concerning computers, minds, and the laws of physics*. Oxford: Oxford University Press; 1989. Print.

Pepler D J. Play and divergent thinking. In: Pepler DJ, Rubin KH. *The Play of Children: current theory and research*. Basel; New York: Karger; 1982. Print.

Pepler DJ, Rubin KH, editors. *The Play of Children: current theory and research*. Basel; New York: Karger; 1982. Print.

Prkachin KM. Dissociating spontaneous and deliberate expressions of pain: signal detection analyses. *Pain*. 1992; **51**(1): 57–65. Print.

Prochaska JO, DiClemente CC. *The Transtheoretical Approach: crossing traditional boundaries of therapy*. Malabar, Florida: R. E. Krieger; 1994. Print.

Proshansky H. The field of environmental psychology. *Handbook of Environmental Psychology*. New York: Wiley; 1987. Print.

Proshansky H, Fabian A, Kaminoff R. Place-identity: physical world socialization of the self. *J Environ Psychol*. 1983; **3**(1): 57–83. Print.

Quakers. *Quaker Faith & Practice: the book of Christian discipline of the yearly meeting of the Religious Society of Friends (Quakers) in Britain*. London: Yearly Meeting of the Religious Society of Friends (Quakers) in Britain; 2009. Print.

Reuler JB, Nardone DA. Role modeling in medical education. *West J Med*. 1994; **160**(4): 335–7. Print.

Rolfe G, Freshwater D, Jasper M. *Critical Reflection for Nursing and the Helping Professions: a user's guide*. Houndmills, Basingstoke, Hampshire: Palgrave; 2001. Print.

Rossman J. *Industrial Creativity; the psychology of the inventor*. New Hyde Park, NY: University; 1964. Print.

Roter DL, Frankel RM, Hall JA, Sluyter D. The expression of emotion through nonverbal behavior in medical visits. Mechanisms and outcomes. *J Gen Intern Med*. 2006; **21**(Suppl. 1): S28–34. Print.

Sackett DL, Rosenberg WM, Gray JA, *et al*. Evidence based medicine: what it is and what it isn't. *BMJ*. 1996; **312**: 71–2. Print.

Sandman, L, Munthe C. Shared decision making, paternalism and patient choice. *Health Care Anal*. 2010; **18**(1): 60–84. Print.

Schegloff EA, Jefferson G, Sacks H. The preference for self-correction in the organization of repair in conversation. *Language*. 1977; **53**: 361–82. Print.

Schön DA. *The Reflective Practitioner: how professionals think in action*. Aldershot: Ashgate; [1983] 2002. Print.

Schwarz, B. *The Paradox of Choice: why more is less*. HarperCollins; New edition; 2005. Print.

Searle JR. *Mind: a brief introduction*. Oxford: Oxford University Press; 2004. Print.

Segal Z, Williams JM, Teasdale J. *Mindfulness-Based Cognitive Therapy for Depression: a new approach to preventing relapse*. New York: Guildford; 2001. Print.

Seligman MEP. *Authentic Happiness: using the new positive psychology to realize your potential for lasting fulfillment*. New York: Free; 2002. Print.

Sharot T, De Martino B, Dolan RJ. Neural activity predicts attitude change in cognitive dissonance. *Nature Neuroscience*. 2009; **29**(12): 3760–5. Print.

Silverman J, Kurtz SM, Draper J. *Skills for Communicating with Patients*. 3rd ed. London: Radcliffe Publishing; 2013. Print.

Simon HA. The mind's eye in chess. In: Chase WG, editor. *Visual Information Processing*. New York: Academic; 1973. Print.

Simon P, Garfunkel A. *The Sounds of Silence*. Columbia, released 1965. CD.

Simonton DK. Creativity, leadership, and chance. In: Sternberg RJ, editor. *The Nature of Creativity*. Cambridge: Cambridge University Press; 1988. Print.

Smith HW. *The 10 Natural Laws of Successful Time and Life Management: proven strategies for increased productivity and inner peace*. New York, NY: Warner; 2003. Print.

Snyder CR, Lopez SJ, editors. *Handbook of Positive Psychology*. Oxford: Oxford University Press; 2009. Print.

Soria R, Legido A, Escolano C. A randomised controlled trial of motivational interviewing for smoking cessation. *Br J Gen Pract*. 2006; **1**(56): 531. Print.

Sowa JF. 'Representing knowledge soup in language and logic'. Available online at: www.jfsowa.com/talks/souprepr.htm

Sternberg RJ. *Beyond IQ: A Triarchic Theory of Intelligence*. Cambridge: Cambridge University Press; 1985.

Stewart I, Joines V. *TA Today: a new introduction to transactional analysis*. Nottingham: Lifespace Pub.; 1987. Print.

Stewart M, Roter D. *Communicating with Medical Patients*. Newbury Park: Sage Publications; 1989. Print.

Stiglitz JE, Sen A, Fitoussi J-P. *Report by the Commission on the Measurement of Economic Performance and Social Progress*. Paris: Commission; 2009. Print.

Stott NC, Davis RH. The exceptional potential in each primary care consultation. *J R Coll Gen Pract*. 1979; **29**: 201–5. Print.

Suzuki DT. *Essays in Zen Buddhism, third series*. London: Published for the Buddhist Society by Rider; 1958. Print.

Suzuki S, Dixon T. *Zen Mind, Beginner's Mind*. New York: Walker/Weatherhill; 1970. Print.

Tarski A. *Logic, Semantics, Metamathematics; papers from 1923 to 1938*. Oxford: Clarendon; 1956. Print.

Taylor D, Bury M. Chronic illness, expert patients and care transition. *Sociology of Health & Illness*. 2007; **29**(1): 27–45. Print.

Tellegen A, Lykken DT, Bouchard TJ, *et al*. Personality similarity in twins reared apart and together. *J Pers Soc Psychol*. 1988; **54**(6): 1031–9. Print.

Thich Nhat Hanh, Mobi Ho, Vo-Dinh Mai. *Miracle of Mindfulness: an introduction*. Boston: Beacon; 1975. Print.

Top Nursing Colleges. *Nursing Theories and Sub-theories*. Top Nursing Colleges. Web. Available at: www.topnursingcolleges.com/nur/nursing-theories-and-sub-theories.html (accessed 12 November 2011).

Tsao L. How much do we know about the importance of play in child development. *Childhood Educ*. Summer 2002. Findarticles.com. Web. Available at: http://findarticles.com/p/articles/mi_qa3614/is_200207/ai_n9147500

Tuckett D, Boulton M, Olson C, Williams A. *Meetings between Experts: an approach to sharing ideas in medical consultations*. London: Tavistock, 1985. Print.

Ubel PA, Angott AM, Zikmund-Fischer BJ. Physicians recommend different treatment for patients than they would choose for themselves. *Arch Intern Med*. 2011; **171**(18): 630–4. Print.

Bibliography

Ulrich RS. How design impacts wellness. *Healthc Forum J.* 1992; **35**(5): 20–5. Print.

Upton J. *Comments.* FearFighter for Panic and Anxiety. Web. Available at: www.fear fighter.com (accessed 28 October 2011).

US National Cancer Institute. *Cancer Screening Overview (PDQ®).* US National Cancer Institute. Web. Available at: www.cancer.gov/cancertopics/pdq/screening/overview/HealthProfessional/page1 (accessed 24 October 2011).

Van Ham I, Verhoeven A, Groenier K, Groothoff J and De Haan J. Job satisfaction among general practitioners: A systematic literature review. *Eur J Gen Pract.* 2006, **12**(4): 174–80. (doi:10.1080/13814780600994376)

Van Veen V, Krug MK, Scooler JW, Carter CS. Neural activity predicts attitude change in cognitive dissonance. *Nature Neuroscience.* 2009; **12**(11): 1469–74. Print.

Vandervert L, Schimpf P, Liu H. How working memory and the cerebellum collaborate to produce creativity and innovation. *Creativity Res J.* 2007; **19**(1): 1–18. Print.

Various. Evidence based practice in clinical hypnosis. *IJCEH.* 2007; **55**(2): n.p. Print.

Walker L. *Consulting with NLP: Neuro-linguistic Programming in the medical consultation.* Oxford: Radcliffe Medical Press; 2002. Print.

Wallas G. *The Art of Thought.* New York: Harcourt, Brace; 1926. Print.

Warren KS. *Coping with the Biomedical Literature: a primer for the scientist and the clinician.* New York, NY: Praeger; 1981. Print.

Waskett C. An integrated approach to introducing and maintaining supervision: the 4S Model. *Nurs Times.* 2009; **105**(17): 24–6. Print.

Weisberg RW. *Creativity: beyond the myth of genius.* New York: W.H. Freeman; 1993. Print.

West C. Against our will: male interruptions of females in cross-sex conversation. *Annals of the New York Academy of Sciences.* 1979 (Language, Sex); **327**(1): 81–96. Print.

White M. *Maps of Narrative Practice.* New York: W.W. Norton & Co; 2007. Print.

White M, Epston D. *Narrative Means to Therapeutic Ends.* New York: Norton; 1990. Print.

Wilber K. *A Brief History of Everything.* Boston, MA: Shambhala; 2007. Print.

Wilber K. An integral theory of consciousness. *J Consciousness Stud.* 1997; **4**(1): 71–92. Print.

Williams CJ, Garland A. Cognitive-behavioural therapy assessment model for use in clinical practice. *Adv Psych Treat.* 2002; **8**: 172–79. Print.

Williams ES, Konrad TR. Physician, practice, and patient characteristics related to primary care physician physical and mental health: results from the Physician Worklife Study. *Health Services Res.* 2002; **37**(1): 119–41. Print.

Williams ES, Konrad TR, Scheckler WE, *et al.* Understanding physicians' intentions to withdraw from practice: the role of job satisfaction, job stress, mental and physical health. *Health Care Manage Rev.* 2010; **35**(2): 105–15. Web.

Wilson PM, Kendall S, Brooks F. The Expert Patients Programme: a paradox of patient empowerment and medical dominance. *Health & Social Care in the Community.* 2007; **15**(5): 426–38. Web.

Yovel G, Kanwisher N. Face perception: domain specific, not process specific. *Neuron.* 2004; **44**(5): 889–98. Print.

Zhong E, Kenward K, Sheets V, *et al.* Probation and recidivism: remediation among disciplined nurses in six states. *Am J Nurs.* 2009; **109**(3): 48–57. Print.

CPD with Radcliffe

You can now use a selection of our books to achieve CPD (Continuing Professional Development) points through directed reading.

We provide a free online form and downloadable certificate for your appraisal portfolio. Look for the CPD logo and register with us at: www.radcliffehealth.com/cpd

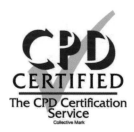